Public Health Issues in Disaster Preparedness

Focus on Bioterrorism

Edited by

Lloyd F. Novick, MD, MPH
Commissioner of Health
Onondaga County, New York
and
Professor
Department of Medicine
SUNY Upstate Medical University
Syracuse, New York

John S. Marr, MD, MPH
Medical Director
Oxford Health Plans
White Plains, New York

JONES AND BARTLETT PUBLISHERS
Sudbury, Massachusetts
BOSTON TORONTO LONDON SINGAPORE

World Headquarters
Jones and Bartlett Publishers
40 Tall Pine Drive
Sudbury, MA 01776
978-443-5000
info@jbpub.com
www.jbpub.com

Jones and Bartlett Publishers Canada
2406 Nikanna Road
Mississauga, ON L5C 2W6
CANADA

Jones and Bartlett Publishers International
Barb House, Barb Mews
London W6 7PA
UK

Originally published by Aspen Publishers, 2001

Adapted from *Journal of Public Health Management and Practice,* Vol. 6:4, ©2000, Aspen Publishers, Inc., and *Public Health Administration: Principles for Population-Based Management,* Lloyd F. Novick, Glen P. Mays, eds., ©2001, Aspen Publishers, Inc.

Production Credits
Chief Executive Officer: Clayton Jones
Chief Operating Officer: Don W. Jones, Jr.
Executive V.P. & Publisher: Robert W. Holland, Jr.
VP, Sales and Marketing: William Kane
Acquisitions Editor: David Cella
Manufacturing Buyer: Amy Bacus

ISBN: 0-7637-2500-5

Printed in the United States of America
07 06 05 04 03 10 9 8 7 6 5 4 3 2 1

Contents

v
INTRODUCTION
LLOYD F. NOVICK
JOHN S. MARR

1
Roles and Responsibilities of Public Health in Disaster Preparedness and Response
LINDA YOUNG LANDESMAN
JOSEPHINE MALILAY
RICHARD A. BISSELL
STEVEN M. BECKER
LES ROBERTS
MICHAEL S. ASCHER

The authors discuss the roles and responsibilities of public health to prepare for and respond to disasters. Carrying out these responsibilities effectively requires a multiorganizational response. Also discussed are the essential roles that public health organizations play in managing the psychological effects of disasters and in managing environmental resources to ensure disaster preparedness.

57
Taking the Terror Out of Bioterrorism: Planning for a Bioterrorist Event from a Local Perspective
LARRY C. GARRETT
CHARLES MAGRUDER
CRAIG A. MOLGARD

The authors argue that because direct support for most public health services, including bioterrorism preparedness, occurs primarily at the local level, this is the logical starting point for all planning activities.

64
Bioterrorism Threats: Learning from Inappropriate Responses
LEONARD A. COLE

Cole describes several recent bioterrorism hoaxes in which emergency responders treated victims inappropriately. He also offers lessons learned from the hoaxes.

75
Bioterrorism: Agents of Concern
THEODORE J. CIESLAK
EDWARD M. EITZEN, JR.

This article highlights the need to have a working knowledge of the diagnosis, pathogenesis, and treatment of the diseases caused by biological agents in the event of a terrorist attack.

85
A History of Biological and Chemical Warfare and Terrorism
CURTIS D. MALLOY

Malloy contends that examining disease in history will provide public health specialists with the knowledge necessary to improve our surveillance system for potential acts of bioterrorism.

93
Bioterrorism: A Challenge to Public Health and Medicine
MARGARET A. HAMBURG

Hamburg provides an overview of the threat of bioterrorism, the roles of public health and medicine, and the critical issues that need to be addressed as the U.S. prepares for potential bioterrorist acts.

99
Bioterrorism Preparedness: Planning for the Future
LISA D. ROTZ
DENISE KOO
PATRICK W. O'CARROLL
RICHARD B. KELLOGG
MICHAEL J. SAGE
SCOTT R. LILLIBRIDGE

Rotz et al. highlight efforts by the CDC and its public health partners to prepare for the threat of biological terrorism.

104
Intergovernmental Preparedness and Response to Potential Catastrophic Biological Terrorism
STEVEN KUHR
JEROME M. HAUER

This article emphasizes enhancing public health and emergency management programs to include preparedness initiatives focused directly on bioweapons surveillance and detection.

111
Bioterrorism: Challenges and Opportunities for Local Health Departments
RICHARD J. GALLO
DYAN CAMPBELL

Gallo and Campbell discuss the need for local and state health departments to work together to develop resources to prepare for potential bioterrorism acts.

117
COMMENTARY
The Role and Responsibility of the Media in the Event of a Bioterrorist Act
HUGH W. WYATT

Wyatt argues that the media must be accurate and responsible in the event of a bioterrorist attack.

121

Internet Resources Related to Biological and Chemical Terrorism

This article highlights some of the top government, nongovernment, and medical/scientific Web sites related to bioterrorism.

123

Public Health Grand Rounds Addresses Bioterrorism Preparedness

WILLIAM L. ROPER
DONNA E. DAVIS

The authors discuss Public Health Grand Rounds, a series of programs on contemporary public health issues aimed at educating health leaders and practitioners.

125

Prioritization Methods for HIV Community Planning

ANA P. JOHNSON-MASOTTI
STEVEN D. PINKERTON
DAVID R. HOLTGRAVE

This article describes and compares four prioritization methods to assist community planning groups in shaping local HIV prevention efforts.

139

Assessing the HIV Prevention Capacity Building Needs of Community-Based Organizations

DONNA L. RICHTER
MARY S. PRINCE
LINDA H. POTTS
BELINDA M. REININGER
MELVA V. THOMPSON
JACQUIE P. FRASER
SUSAN L. FULMER

The authors discuss a cross-sectional survey of community-based organizations conducted to assess a variety of training issues that would benefit their HIV prevention services.

Introduction

The threat of bioterrorism has been highlighted by the September 11th attack on the World Trade Center. This tragedy raises understandable concerns that other methods of attack, biological and chemical, now have increased likelihood. There is a new public mandate to increase our preparedness. A strong and effective public health infrastructure is essential for the surveillance and recognition of microbial and other hazards. Modes to enhance communication and coordination of many community entities in emergency situations are required. Foremost is the role that must be played by local health departments in leading the surveillance, risk reduction and response efforts. Public health agencies are on the frontlines in dealing with this new reality as well as coping with hoaxes, rumors, public perceptions and fear.

The contents of this volume are essential to all of those concerned with public health and safety. This special report combines an issue of the *Journal of Public Health Management and Practice* focused on bioterrorism (Issue Editor, John Marr) and a chapter from the recently published book *Public Health Administration: Principles for Population-Based Management*, "Roles and Responsibilities of Public Health in Disaster Preparedness and Response (lead author, Linda Landesman)." Its recommendations are detailed and experience-based. The technical aspects of bioterrorism agents are outlined and the planning and communication elements necessary to reduce the risk to our population are described. Authorities contributing to these works are experts at the national, state and local levels. Contributors include those involved in the remarkable planning done in New York City to address these problems. Environmental, Emergency Medical Services and protocols for disaster response are included. Importantly, as demonstrated by the recent event, attention to the mental health concomitants of disaster are addressed in detail.

The technological know-how to produce and deliver bioterrotist weapons is limited by production, storage and dissemination obstacles. However, the threat of this hazard is a reality and the potential impact is devastating. Surveillance, identification, planning and preparedness are required. Building the capacity of local public health agencies as leaders of this effort is now a priority. This document outlines the fundamentals required for all communities.

Lloyd F. Novick, MD, MPH
John S. Marr, MD, MPH

Roles and Responsibilities of Public Health in Disaster Preparedness and Response

Linda Young Landesman, Josephine Malilay, Richard A. Bissell, Steven M. Becker, Les Roberts, and Michael S. Ascher

Public health has broad responsibilities to prepare for and respond to disasters. Carrying out these responsibilities effectively requires a multiorganizational response. Key among these responsibilities are disaster epidemiology and assessment, which are used as managerial tools as well as instruments of scientific investigation. Public health organizations also play essential roles in managing the psychosocial effects of disasters and in managing environmental resources to ensure disaster preparedness. The emerging threat of bioterrorism creates new risks and responsibilities for public health organizations. Although the challenges of managing environmental health threats are greater in developing countries than in the United States, essential elements of public health administration—including the management of food, water, and waste—can be compromised substantially in the most devastating domestic disasters, creating imperatives for disaster preparedness.

DISASTERS HAVE BEEN defined as ecologic disruptions, or emergencies, of a severity and magnitude resulting in deaths, injuries, illness, and/or property damage that cannot be effectively managed by the application of routine procedures or resources and that result in a call for outside assistance. As the field of disaster study evolved, a common set of vocabulary emerged as well, notably distinguishing among hazards, emergencies, and disasters.[1]

- *Hazards* present the probability of the occurrence of a disaster caused by a natural phenomenon (e.g., earthquake, tropical cyclone), by failure of manmade sources of energy (e.g., nuclear reactor,

Linda Young Landesman, DrPH, MSW, *is Assistant Vice President at the Office of Professional Services and Affiliations of the New York City Health and Hospitals Corporation in New York, New York.*

Josephine Malilay, PhD, MPH, *is an Epidemiologist at the Health Studies Branch in the Division of Environmental Hazards and Health Effects at the Centers for Disease Control and Prevention in Atlanta, Georgia.*

Richard A. Bissell, PhD, *is Associate Professor in the Department of Emergency Health Services at the University of Maryland Baltimore County in Baltimore, Maryland.*

Steven M. Becker, JD, CPA, *is Executive Director of the Association of Public Health Laboratories in Washington, DC.*

Les Roberts, PhD, MSPH, *is a Lecturer at Whiting School of Engineering at The Johns Hopkins University in Baltimore, Maryland.*

Michael S. Ascher, MD, FACP, *is Chief of the Viral and Richettsial Disease Laboratory in the Division of Communicable Disease Control at the California Department of Health Services in Berkeley, California.*

industrial explosion), or by uncontrolled human activity (e.g., conflicts, overgrazing).

- *Emergencies* are typically any occurrence that requires an immediate response.[1] These events can be the result of nature (e.g., hurricanes, tornados, and earthquakes), can be caused by technological or manmade error (e.g., nuclear accidents, bombing, and bioterrorism), or can be the result of emerging diseases (e.g., West Nile virus in New York City).
- *Natural disasters* suggest rapid, acute onset phenomena (sudden-onset events) with profound effects, such as earthquakes, floods, tropical cyclones, and tornadoes. *Manmade disasters,* also called complex emergencies, suggest technological events or disasters that are not caused by natural hazards but that occur in human settlements, such as fire, chemical spills and explosions, and armed conflict. No clear demarcation exists between the two categories. For instance, fire may be the result of arson, a manmade activity, but may also occur secondarily to earthquake events, particularly in urban areas where gas mains may be damaged. With increasing technological development worldwide, a new category of disasters known as *natural–technological, or "na-tech," disasters,* has been described in the literature. Na-tech disasters refer to natural disasters that create technological emergencies, such as urban fires resulting from seismic motion or chemical spills resulting from floods.[2]

The life cycle of a disaster event is typically known as the disaster continuum, or emergency management cycle. Before (preimpact), during (impact), and after (postimpact) a disaster event, both public health and emergency management officials and the population at risk can reduce or prevent injury, illness, or death by the actions they take. The basic phases of disaster management include mitigation or prevention, warning and preparedness, response and recovery. *Mitigation* includes the measures that are taken to reduce the harmful effects of a disaster by attempting to limit impacts on human health and economic infrastructure. Although prevention may refer to preventing a disaster from occurring, such as cloud seeding to stimulate rain in fire situations, in public health terms, *prevention* refers to actions that may prevent further loss of life, disease, disability, or injury. *Warning* or forecasting refers to the monitoring of events to look for indicators that signify when and where a disaster might occur and what the magnitude might be. In *preparedness,* officials or the public itself structure a response to disasters that may occur and, in so doing, lay the framework for recovery.

In the United States, the *response* to disasters is organized through multiple jurisdictions, agencies, and authorities. The term "emergency management" is used to refer to these activities. The emergency management field organizes its activities by "sectors" such as fire, police, and emergency medical services (EMS). The response phase of a disaster encompasses relief and is followed by recovery and rehabilitation or reconstruction. *Emergency relief* focuses attention on saving lives, providing first aid, restoring emergency communications and transportation systems, and providing immediate care and basic needs to survivors, such as food and clothing or medical and emotional care. *Recovery* includes actions for returning the community to normal, such as repairing infrastructure, damaged buildings, and critical facilities. *Rehabilitation* or *reconstruction* involves activities that are taken to counter the effects of the disaster on long-term development.[3]

Domestically, there are 40–50 presidential disaster declarations per year. The Stafford Act, passed by Congress in 1988, provides for orderly assistance by the federal government to state and local governments to help them to carry out their responsibilities in managing major disasters and emergencies.[4] A disaster declaration must precede any federal aid whereby states make a request for federal assistance to activate a declaration. Most presidential declarations are made immediately following impact. However, if the consequences of a disaster are imminent and warrant limited predeployment actions to lessen or avert the threat of a catastrophe, a state's governor may submit a request even before the disaster has occurred. Although rarely used, the president may exercise his authority in certain emergencies and make a disaster declaration prior to state request in order to expedite the sending of federal resources. This presidential authority was used immediately following the 1995 bombing in Oklahoma City. Under the Stafford Act, the president may provide federal resources, medicine, food and other consumables, work and services, and financial assistance.

Disasters pose a number of unique health care problems that have little counterpart in the routine practice of emergency health care. Examples include the need for warning and evacuation of residents, widespread "urban" search and rescue, triage and distribution of casualties, having to function within a damaged or disabled health care infrastructure, and coordination among multiple jurisdictions, among levels of government, and among private sector organizations. In order to be effective managers, public health professionals must be knowledgeable about unfamiliar information such as the lexicon of emergency management and the science of engineering and must be competent in a specialized set of skills because disasters pose unique health care problems. For example, although temporary deficiencies in resources may occur at certain times in any disaster, resource problems in U.S. disasters more often relate to how assets are used or distributed rather than to deficiencies.[5] In a study of the impact of 29 major mass casualty disasters on hospitals, only six percent of the involved hospitals had supply shortages, and only two percent had personnel shortages.[6]

Why Public Health Should Be Concerned

Public health professionals should augment their ability to respond to disasters for the following reasons:

- The occurrence of natural disasters is increasing.
- There is a ubiquitous risk across the United States.
- Disasters have negative impacts on health.
- The effects of disasters will escalate, generating an increased need for public health intervention.
- Public health has the expertise to help communities handle the most common health-related problems.

Across the globe, mankind is experiencing an increase in natural disasters, as evidenced by events in recent years.[7,8] Once a week, an average of one disaster that requires external international assistance occurs somewhere in the world. On a worldwide average, approximately 81,000 people die from natural disasters yearly. In the last two decades, as a consequence of disasters, more than 1.620 million people died, 3.5 billion lives were disrupted, and $900 billion was lost in property damage.[9]

Natural Disasters

Residents of the United States share a ubiquitous risk.[10] Across the United States, a massive number of people are at risk from three classes of natural disasters: floods, earthquakes, and hurricanes. There are more than 6,000 communities with populations of 2,500 or more persons located in flood plains that have been highly developed as living and working environments.[11] At least 70 million people face significant risk of death or injury from earthquakes because they live in the 39 states that are seismically active. In California alone, if a single major earthquake occurs, similar to nine others that occurred in the state over the past 150 years, there could be 20,000 deaths, 100,000 injuries, and economic losses totaling more than $100 billion.[12] Other parts of the country face serious risk because more than 3 million people live within a 75-mile radius of the New Madrid fault in the Midwest.[13] Even in Utah, there is a 20 percent probability that a large earthquake of a magnitude of 7.5 will occur on some segment of the Wasatch front within the next 50 years.[14]

Currently, 110 million people live in coastal areas of the United States, including the Great Lakes region. By the year 2010, the coastal population will have grown from 80 million people in 1960 to more than 127 million people—an increase of 60 percent nationwide.[15] The significance of this shift is evident when the risk posed by hurricanes alone is examined. Because of climatic changes in western Africa, hurricane activity along the Atlantic Coast and the Gulf of Mexico is expected to become as frequent as that which occurred between 1940–50.[8] During that decade, three category 4–5 hurricanes struck Miami, New Orleans, and the Gulf Coast. Since 1989, three category 4 hurricanes (Hugo, Andrew, and Opal) struck the East Coast of the United States from Florida to New England. A category 4 or greater hurricane crosses the U.S. coastline nearly once every six years.

Disasters have negative impacts on the public's health. These events result in increases in morbidity and mortality, with both physical and psychological impacts that could be reduced with adequate intervention. Following the 1993 floods in the Midwest, victims increased their use of primary health care and experienced long-term impediments to their access to health care.[16] Local health departments

(LHDs) in Missouri understood the need for involvement in preparedness efforts because they experienced difficulties in collecting and using assessment information, coordination was burdensome, and there were interorganizational impediments to an effective response.[17]

Manmade Disasters

Manmade or technological disasters can also have devastating impacts on the public's health. The 1992 civil unrest in Los Angeles caused 53 deaths, more than 2,000 injuries, and destruction or closure to 15 county health centers, 45 pharmacies, and 38 medical and dental offices. There were also significant impacts to the quality of water, to hazardous materials and solid waste, and to protecting sources of food.[18] Because widespread burning, as occurred in the civil unrest, can release hazardous materials into the air, almost 3,000 sites were surveyed for release of hazardous waste.[18]

The actual and potential effects of manmade disasters will likely escalate, generating an increased need for public health intervention as the world's population grows, as population density increases, and as technology becomes more sophisticated. The need for public health information has spurred the development of readily available guidance. The National Center for Environmental Health at the U.S. Centers for Disease Control and Prevention (CDC) developed preventive guidelines, available on the CDC Web site, promoting personal health and safety for people involved in earthquakes, floods, hurricanes, and tornadoes.[19] High mortality attributed to the 1995 heat wave in Chicago demonstrated the need for standardized methodologies to make comparisons across geographic areas of the country.[20]

Public Health Personnel

Worldwide, the growing number of humanitarian emergencies has resulted in an expanding need for skilled public health professionals. The application of public health principles in a domestic response differs from public health practice in an international response, but the competencies required of the profession are the same. The tasks involved in fostering the development of community self-sufficiency are also functionally different in the United States than in international development. In developed countries, the medical response for emergency care is well organized through EMS. In developing countries, that infrastructure doesn't exist. In developing countries, public health personnel often play a key role because virtually all of the problems are related to the health of the populations. In complex humanitarian emergencies, public health personnel:

- Conduct initial assessments of health needs.
- Design and establish health activities.
- Plan for the delivery of services.
- Establish refugee camps.
- Provide and monitor food supplies.
- Supervise and monitor environmental health activities.
- Monitor the protection of human rights.

Public health can help communities handle the most common health-related problems. There are four domains where public health expertise is superior to that of other professionals involved in disaster preparedness and response. Public health officials are trained to conduct *assessments,* to survey the impacted site and determine the scope of damage and subsequent impacts on the community and the population. Using the management information systems that public health officials have developed throughout the health care industry, public health professionals are well prepared to *share information.* Some creative fine-tuning will permit public health professionals to develop procedures for capturing and sharing disaster-related information among the health community and other response organizations. Public health can build on the *triage* procedures used in emergency medicine to help other responders prioritize both medical and public health problems. Finally, public health's knowledge of *casualty distribution* will facilitate the development of procedures for disbursing casualties among available hospitals.

Disaster preparedness poses the quintessential public health dilemma—how to motivate people to prevent disaster-related health problems. It is human nature to say that "a major disaster will never happen here" and to fail to prepare. Health care organizations often don't give high priority to preparing for disastrous events, which are rare, when the general financial environment for health care is fragile. Furthermore, the benefits of preparedness often are not evident until after a disaster has occurred. In addition, economic constraints are often coupled with public apathy. Social scientists have noted that the public's perception of risk is often not correlated with actual risk, and that risks are usually downplayed. Many people continue to live in flood plains, even after repeated floods, and millions of people move to areas that are located on earthquake faults.

However, the benefits of effective prevention are demonstrated in a comparison of the morbidity and mortality statistics of Hurricane Andrew (Florida,1992) and the hurricane that struck, without warning, off the Gulf Coast of Texas in 1900. Due to successful prediction, warning, and evacuation, actual deaths following Andrew were less than two dozen. By contrast, in Texas 90 years earlier, 6,000 people were killed and 5,000 were injured.[21] Because of strong planning, the Los Angeles Department of Health provided important services following the 1994 Northridge earthquake.[22] Public health intervened when there were concerns about water and sewage, provided assessments of personal and mental health, inspected health care facilities, restored clinical operations, and educated the public about safety, health, and environmental concerns.

History of Public Health's Role

Although public health is late in contributing to disaster preparedness and response, epidemiology made an early contribution to the domain of disaster research. Noji detailed the course of epidemiology's research contribution.[23] In 1957, Saylor and Gordon suggested using epidemiologic parameters to define disasters.[24] Almost a decade later, the CDC helped develop techniques for the rapid assessment of nutritional status in Nigeria. The 1970s brought the establishment of the Centre for Research on Epidomiology of Disasters in Belgium and specialized units within the World Health Organization (WHO) and the Pan American Health Organization (PAHO). The science of public health has now begun to show that variations in morbidity and mortality from one country to another are often due to differences in building standards and population density rather than the magnitude of an earthquake. This is demonstrated by a comparison of the impacts of recent hurricanes. In California, where antiseismic building and land use codes are well enforced, the Northridge earthquake of 1994 resulted in 57 deaths and almost 9,200 serious injuries.[22] In contrast, in Armenia, with poor construction and antiseismic regulations insufficient and poorly enforced, an earthquake of lesser magnitude killed 25,000 people and injured more than 100,000. The August 1999 earthquake in Turkey resulted in a variable rate of collapse of buildings that were built side by side. The standards used for construction were the determinate factor for a structure's survival.

The earliest investigations of disaster response were conducted by sociologists who studied organizational behavior under stress. Other contributions have been made by psychologists, management scientists, architects, engineers, economists, and public administrators. Since the early 1980s, there has been increased attention and interest in organizing a public health response to disasters and conducting studies within the public health discipline. The eruption of Mt. St. Helens in 1980 accelerated the involvement of the U.S. federal government in organizing a response.[25,26] The United Nations (UN) declared the 1990s as the disaster decade, International Decade for Natural Disaster Reduction, due to continued human losses across the globe.[27] The declaration for the decade spurred a broad variety of academic disciplines to develop educational and research programs in all phases of disaster management. The decade came to an end on December 31, 1999, and was succeeded by the International Strategy for Disaster Reduction as adopted by resolution 54/219 of the General Assembly of the UN.[28]

Historically, public health's response to disasters has been an ad hoc one, and on the whole, the profession has reacted slower than other disciplines in organizing professional activities. In many locales across the country, the medical/health efforts of preparedness have not been coordinated as part of the community's disaster response. Health departments were called in as an afterthought to handle problems that were part of their domain, rather than as part of the team planning the response. Other professions, such as emergency medicine, EMS, and engineering, increased training earlier in the decade to prepare their membership better for responding to disasters. The medical literature regarding disasters is full of anecdotal accounts of response.[5] However, few of these reports substantiate the *effectiveness* of the reported preparedness.

Public Health's Role

Public health has a natural role in disaster preparedness and response. This role is evolving as the emergency management community recognizes the skills possessed by the profession. Through increased recognition of what public health professionals can do, public health professionals are being called on more often to control injury and disease that are caused by both natural and technological hazards and to prevent infectious disease following natural disasters. State departments of health, with responsibility as a major directing unit overseeing the public's health, already work in partnership with LHDs and other appropriate federal, state, and local agencies. Disaster response is often an extension of daily tasks for public health professionals. In many states and localities, public health professionals coordinate the health response following natural and technological emergencies.[29]

Due to its impact on realms where public health is core, including health care infrastructure, Hurricane Andrew demonstrated that public health professionals must be involved in preparedness and response operations. Following Hurricane Andrew, which was categorized as "the most destructive disaster ever to affect the United States,"[30(p.243)] 175,000 Floridians were homeless and water systems were inoperable for at least a week.[21] The infrastructure of the health care system was also destroyed—59 hospitals were damaged, more than 12,000 patients needed to be examined, and pharmacies couldn't dispense medication.[31] To help in this situation, more than 850 public health nurses were deployed during the two months following the storm.[32]

With the increase in both domestic natural disasters and international complex emergencies, there is greater recognition of the need for intergovernmental experts who understand disasters. Although the calls for widespread training of the public health work force began relatively recently, there is now mainstream recognition that public health is a key player in disaster preparedness and response.[32] *Healthy People 2010* will include, as part of the core competencies, the enhancement of professional training in preparing for and responding to disasters.[33] Federal recognition of the need for public health intervention has resulted in newly directed federal funding at the end of the millennium for departments of health to improve their core abilities to respond to acts of bioterrorism, bringing public health intervention into the core of disaster preparedness and response.

What Is Public Health's Responsibility in Disaster Response?

The mission of public health in disaster preparedness and response includes responsibility for the following domains, referred to as "functions" within the emergency management field:

- assessment of the viability of the health care infrastructure, including the drug supply
- assessment of environmental infrastructure (food, water, sanitation, and vector control)
- assessment and provision of health care services (acute, continuity of care, primary care, and emergency care)
- preventive care
- assessment of the needs of the elderly and other special populations
- health surveillance and case identification/verification, including injury surveillance
- infectious disease control
- expert assistance in response to chemical, radiologic, or biologic hazards
- public health information
- mental health
- emergency shelter
- victim identification/body management

To fulfill these functions, public health has three major tasks.

- One task is the collection, evaluation, and dissemination of information. The other sectors that have traditionally responded to disasters are response oriented, not science oriented. Public health brings a basis for evaluating activities using a scientific method. Public health brings unique resources to the emergency management community. These include assessment and epidemiology and the capacity to analyze, make recommendations, and act on information. As an example, using Stafford Act funds, the state of Iowa established a statewide systematic electronic system for surveillance during the 1993 flood.[34]
- The second task is one of cooperation and collaboration with other disciplines. The responsibilities of public health in disaster preparedness and response are more complicated than in a typical public health response. First, the participants are from "sectors of response" (i.e., fire,

EMS, emergency management) rather than from other parts of the health care delivery field. Workers have to participate as part of a multidisciplinary team that includes mostly professionals or paraprofessionals with whom they normally don't have interactions and who have little or no knowledge of public health (i.e., engineering, police, and the military/national guard). Further, the process of working together is unique. The other sectors who are involved in disaster response have a lexicon and methods that may be different than those of public health. A typical response incorporates multiple bureaucratic layers of infrastructure working together in a condensed time frame. Public health must often integrate itself into an already established response team whose members have trained together and who have clearly defined roles.

- The third task constitutes the prevention of disease and continuity of care. Public health looks at localities where a disaster has occurred, or is likely to occur, as a diseased or compromised community. No other discipline assesses how or acts to prevent disease following disaster. Public health has a major responsibility in ensuring the continuation of the delivery of all health care.

Being prepared is necessitated not only because of legal mandates, but also because of the devastating consequences if health care systems are unable to function. The Joint Commission on Accreditation of Healthcare Organizations prescribes standards and requirements that health care facilities must meet in order to remain accredited. These standards ensure that basic disaster plans are in place and that exercises of these plans are held on a regular basis.[35] The public health professional is involved in ensuring that essential health facilities are able to function after the impact of a disaster.[5,29] Essential facilities include hospitals, health departments, poison control centers, storage sites for disaster supplies, dispatch centers, paging services, and ambulance stations. The maintenance and continuation of home-based services (e.g., dialysis, intravenous antibiotics, visiting nurses services, etc.) will require creative solutions, worked out in advance. Patients in all residential care facilities (long-term care, psychiatric, rehabilitation) may need to be evacuated and placed elsewhere. Public health also initiates arrangements to ensure that routine sources of medical care will be functioning after a disaster. When physicians' offices, mental health clinics, nursing homes, pharmacies, community clinics, and urgent care centers are closed, those individuals needing routine care or medication will seek care from emergency departments based in already stressed hospitals. Following Hurricane Andrew, for example, more than 1,000 physicians' offices were destroyed or significantly damaged, greatly adding to the patient load of surviving hospitals.[32]

Functional Model of Public Health's Response in Disasters

In disaster preparedness and response, public health professionals are providers of service, scientists, and administrators. The core functions of public health have specific application to the organizational model of disaster preparedness and response, providing an opportunity for the breadth of the public health discipline to participate. In order to enter as full members of the emergency management response team, public health practitioners need to relate the framework of activities defined by the emergency management community to what public health can do. In order to provide technical assistance to communities, public health professionals must expand their lexicon to include specialized information that may not be directly related to health and seek out modalities for accessing state-of-the-art resources of other scientific fields, such as earth science, engineering, and demography. This interface between the core components of professional training and the matrix of emergency management is called the functional model of public health's response in disasters.

The functional model provides a paradigm for identifying disaster-related activities for which each core area of public health has responsibility. The functional model is composed of six phases that correspond to the type of activities involved in preparing for and responding to a disaster. The model (Table 1) identifies the roles and tasks for each of the core areas in each phase of a typical disaster response. This paradigm operationalizes a typical disaster response and categorizes the cycle of activities performed by the public health field. The functional

Table 1

Functional model of public health responsibilities in disaster management

	Health administration	Epidemiology/ Biostatistics	Behavioral/ Social sciences	Environment	International
Planning	• Apply local public health to disaster management • Coordinate with hospital disaster plans • Help develop community disaster plan • Provide training • Determine assets	• Provide training • Analyze hazards and vulnerability • Conduct needs assessment	• Develop health promotion and disease prevention • Conduct training	• Conduct training • Analyze hazards and vulnerability	• Analyze hazards and vulnerability and develop response
Prevention Primary	• Provide immunizations • Protect and distribute food • Establish safe water and sanitation		• Educate community • Train public in first aid	• Protect and distribute food • Establish safe water and sanitation	• Provide emergency nutrition • Protect and distribute food • Establish safe water and sanitation
Prevention Secondary	• Detect and extricate victims • Provide emergency care • Manage bystander response		• Detect and extricate • Provide emergency care • Manage bystander response	• Detect and extricate • Provide emergency care • Manage bystander response	
Prevention Tertiary	• Reestablish health services • Manage emergency services • Manage injuries	• Conduct care identification and surveillance • Implement infectious disease control	• Provide long-term counseling		• Convert reponse to development

continues

Table 1

Continued

	Health administration	Epidemiology/ Biostatistics	Behavioral/ Social sciences	Environment	International
Assessments	• Conduct surveillance for disease, behavioral, social, and political impacts • Assess damage to health care infrastructure • Survey assets • Conduct vulnerability analysis • Collect data for decision making	• Conduct surveillance for disease, social, behavioral, and political impacts • Assess causal factors of disease • Conduct vulnerability analysis • Conduct needs assessment • Collect data for decision making • Establish continuous monitoring	• Conduct surveillance for disease, social, behavioral, and political impacts • Collect data for decision making	• Conduct surveillance for disease, social, behavioral, and political impacts • Identify hazards and assess exposure • Conduct vulnerability analysis • Assess damage from: radiation, toxins, thermal, and water • Collect data for decision making • Do short-term cluster sampling • Establish continuous monitoring	• Conduct surveillance for disease, social, behavioral, and political impacts • Collect data for decision making • Do short-term cluster sampling
Service Response	• Administer logistics • Establish command and control, including casualty management • Identify, contain, and provide emergency treatment • Continue provision of primary care • Utilize the Federal Response Plan		• Educate to prevent illness and injury • Organize mental health services	• Identify, contain, and provide emergency equipment	• Utilize international disaster relief, United Nations agencies, International Committee of the Red Cross, and nongovernmental organizations

continues

Table 1

Continued

	Health administration	Epidemiology/ Biostatistics	Behavioral/ Social sciences	Environment	International
Management Response	• Establish infection control, safe water, sanitation, and quarantine • Manage dead, biologic hazards, and waste disposal • Manage media • Utilize field skills • Establish security and protection	• Determine risk of delayed effects • Communicate risk	• Establish information systems	• Establish infection and vector control, safe water, sanitation, and quarantine • Reduce postdisaster injury (fire, nails, and electrocution) • Manage dead, biologic hazards, waste disposal • Communicate risk	• Manage dead, biologic hazards, waste disposal
Surveillance	• Establish information systems	• Utilize information systems • Look for sentinel events • Develop passive and active systems • Establish disaster informatics • Trend disease	• Establish information systems		• Monitor malnutrition
Recovery	• Use data for deployment of resources • Conduct evaluations • Plan and direct fieldwork	• Conduct evaluations • Plan and direct field studies	• Conduct evaluations • Plan and direct field studies	• Conduct evaluations • Plan and direct field studies	• Use data for deployment of resources • Conduct evaluations • Plan and direct fieldwork
Development					• Build capacity • Mobilize resources • Distribute food • Control injury and communicable disease • Provide population-based immunization • Provide primary health care, reproductive health, and transcultural care

Source: Copyright © 2000, L. Landesman.

model expands traditional public health partnerships with other disciplines because it requires public health professionals to collaborate with other responding sectors and to work in an integrated fashion with networks whose roles are previously well defined. The public health role for international scenarios has been independently assessed and described as if it were a conceptual fifth core area.

The components of the model follow:

- *Planning:* The goals of planning are to learn to work cooperatively with other disciplines and understand the resources, skills, and tools that public health professionals bring to the diseased community.
- *Prevention:* Prevention involves primary, secondary, and tertiary efforts and includes the activities that are commonly thought of as "mitigation" in the emergency management model.
- *Assessment:* Assessments are both short-term and long-term snapshots that help with decision making and enhance the profession's ability to monitor disaster situations. The goal of conducting assessments is to convey information quickly in order to recalibrate a system's response.
- *Response:* Response includes both the delivery of services and the management of activities.
- *Surveillance:* Surveillance includes both data collection and monitoring of disease.
- *Recovery:* Recovery has policy, political, and social implications that are both short and long term. Hurricane Floyd (1999) destroyed communities in New Jersey that had never experienced flooding. Many citizens were uninsured and received limited financial aid, making any recovery prolonged and painful.

Structure and Organizational Makeup of Disaster Response

When the health care sector responds to a disaster, it is most efficient to do so with the resources already at hand. However, because disasters overwhelm the local authority's ability to respond effectively in protecting human health, local assets often need to be supplemented by resources from outside organizations. Additionally, disasters typically generate needs that are beyond the breadth of any one type of health care organization. This tension between need and availability is overcome by planning for and mounting a *multiorganizational* response, one of the key characteristics of disaster operations in the health sector. This section provides a quick overview of the organizations that are typically involved in the health sector's response to disaster, and describes how they interact with each other in disaster situations. Table 2 provides a listing of the most important response organizations.

Structure and Operations of the Routine EMS System

For most sudden-onset disasters, the first medical response is provided by the local or regional EMS system. The EMS system constitutes a portion of the health care delivery system that is virtually unknown to many public health professionals. Although its public health role in routine crisis management is beyond the scope of this chapter, the potential public health impact that can be contributed by EMS in times of disaster is substantial.[36] For this reason, it is important for public health emergency planners to be familiar with the organization and operations of the EMS system in both routine and disaster configurations.

In most parts of the United States, EMS is provided by semiautonomous local agencies with regional or state oversight. This service is provided under the authority of the state health department in most, but not all, states, but is not provided directly by the health department. EMS is thought to consist of

- a *public access system* by which the public notifies authorities that a medical emergency exists (In most of the United States, the 911 emergency telephone system is the backbone of this public access.)
- a *dispatch communications system* by which ambulance personnel and other emergency first responders are dispatched to respond to the person(s) in need
- *trained emergency medical responders*, commonly called emergency medical technicians (EMTs), or the higher-trained Paramedics (EMT-Ps) (EMTs and paramedics are trained to identify and field treat the most common medical emergencies and injuries, and to provide medical support to victims while they are enroute to the hospital.)
- *transportation* to definitive medical care, usually in a hospital (Ground ambulances are the

Table 2

Disaster response organizations

Organization	Functions and definitions
Public Access System	Enables public to communicate response needs, typically through a 911 phone system.
Fire Department	Finds and extricates victims; often provides on-scene incident management.
Emergency Medical Services (EMS)	Assesses scene for medical needs, initiates triage of patients, assesses individual patients for status and treatment needs, initiates life-sustaining first aid and medical care, determines treatment destination, and transports patients to definitive care.
Incident Management System (IMS or ICS)	This is a *function*, often provided by an emergency management agency, a fire department, or multiple agencies.
Emergency Management Agency (EMA)	A state or jurisdictional agency tasked with preparedness and response for disasters and other emergencies. This is sometimes called the Office of Emergency Preparedness (OEP).
Federal Emergency Management Agency (FEMA)	The coordinating agency for all federal-level agency responses to disasters.
American Red Cross (ARC)	Private voluntary national organization tasked by government to provide mass care and shelter to disaster victims.
U.S. Public Health Services (USPHS)	The federal action agency charged with protecting the public's health.
Emergency Support Function 8 (ESF 8)	The health and medical function of the Federal Emergency Plan, which is coordinated by the USPHS Office of Emergency Preparedness.
National Disaster Medical System (NDMS)	A multi-agency response system coordinated by the USPHS-OEP with responsibility for responding to overwhelming medical needs in a disaster-struck state or territory.
Disaster Medical Assistance Team (DMAT)	A trained unit of medical response personnel available to respond with the NDMS to a disaster scene.
Private Voluntary Organization (PVO)	A broad range of functions and structures.
Substance Abuse and Mental Health Services Administration (SAMHSA)	One of the eight agencies of the USPHS; focuses on substance abuse and mental health services.
Center for Mental Health Services (CMHS)	Part of the SAMHSA; leads federal efforts to promote mental health and treat mental illness.
Emergency Services and Disaster Relief Branch (ESDRB)	Part of the CMHS; works with other agencies to provide crisis counseling and education to survivors of presidentially declared disasters.
Centers for Disease Control and Prevention (CDC)	
National Center for Environmental Health (NCEH)	Part of the CDC; assesses needs of people in disaster stricken areas and works to ensure that people receive appropriate assistance; has major responsibility for disaster epidemiology.

vehicle of choice for most transports, but helicopters, boats, and snow cats may be used under specific circumstances. Ambulances allow for the continued medical support of patients while in transport.)

- *definitive care*, usually initiated in a hospital emergency department and followed up in a variety of health care settings (Emergency physicians and certified emergency nurses are specialists in emergency medical care in the hospital setting.)

The EMS is often discussed in terms of the prehospital system (e.g., public access, dispatch, EMTs/medics, and ambulance services) and the in-hospital system (e.g., emergency departments, inpatient care, and other definitive care facilities and personnel).

Several designs exist for the organizing authority of prehospital EMS systems: fire service, third service, private, public utility, rescue squad, and hospital based. Somewhat more than half of all EMS systems in the United States are based in local fire departments, with ambulance and fire services administered side by side.[37] In some systems, EMTs or medics are cross-trained as fire fighters with victim extrication skills, and fire fighters are cross-trained as medics. Third service systems are owned and operated by a city or county and are not run by either the fire services or the police service, therefore making them a third service. Some jurisdictions contract with private ambulance services, and some contract with a single private operator on a monopoly basis, which is called a public utility model. In some parts of eastern United States and in many rural areas, EMS is provided by volunteer independent rescue squads, or volunteer ambulance squads that are attached to a volunteer fire department. Finally, some EMS is based in local hospitals, from which they are dispatched and return. In most states, the health department has training and regulation jurisdiction over all EMS personnel regardless of their organizational affiliation. Regardless of the organizational affiliation, all EMS services work in close cooperation with fire department and specialized hazardous material teams to provide patient extrication from entrapment and dangerous situations.

The kind of medical care provided by EMS is divided into basic and advanced life support. The great majority of EMS providers are trained at the basic life support level. Basic life support prepares for the provision of fairly sophisticated noninvasive first aid and stabilization for a broad variety of emergency conditions, as well as semiautomatic defibrillation for cardiac arrest victims. Advanced life support, provided by paramedics, includes sophisticated diagnosis of patient conditions followed by initial on-site, protocol-driven medical treatment for conditions that will receive definitive treatment in hospitals. Paramedics work with a standardized pharmacopia that includes cardiac, respiratory, and blood pressure–related drugs, as well as high-potency short-acting anesthetics and analgesics. Specialized skills include endotracheal intubation, IV cannulation, surgical cricothyrotomy, intraosseous infusion, needle thoracostomy, manual defibrillation, pacing, and cardioversion.

In responding to a disaster, the function of coordinating and managing the multiple simultaneous activities, as well as managing the effective deployment of incoming resources, is of primary importance. Drabek et al. found that the coordination of multiple activities, resource inputs, and organizations was among the most difficult and crucial challenges in managing a disaster response.[38] A strong command and coordination system is imperative if emergency health services are to overcome the disruption to the normal operations of the system and to manage additional incoming resources. First published as the FIRESCOPE Program in 1982, the Incident Command System (alternatively called Incident Management System [IMS]) has become popular among fire services and EMS as a management structure that is able to maintain effective span of control, modular organization, and expandability.[39] Through a system called "sectorization," the tasks and functions of those responding, and the use of resources, are divided into manageable components. As the size or type of the operation changes, it is those sectors that allow for the IMS to be universally applied. Because of this, the IMS has become the standard operating methodology in EMS disaster response.

Organization of Public Health Emergency Response

The basis for all local public health emergency responses resides in the LHD. However, the public health sector is not nearly as uniformly organized for emergency responses as the EMS system is, with its broad variety of system designs. Although some health departments have the emergency response functions preplanned and assigned to appropriate departments, some have only designated someone to function as the emergency coordinator, and others assume that the director or his or her designee will cover any emergency contingencies. The best prepared health departments have well-designed emergency or disaster response plans, complete with a thorough risk analysis, prognostication of probable health effects, and analysis of the resources needed (and available) to provide an appropriate response. The health departments that are well prepared are likely to have coordinated their plans with other response functions in the health sector (EMS and hospitals), and with other public safety efforts, including the IMS. Regrettably, the majority of LHDs are unlikely to have comprehensive disaster response plans that are integrated with other medical response and public safety agencies.

The public health response to local-level emergencies and disasters is inevitably a multidisciplinary effort. The American Red Cross (ARC) provides emergency shelter; basic health services for those residing in shelters; food services on-site and in shelters; counseling, including mental health services or referrals; and family reunification. The public works department or a contracted commercial provider most often manages the potable water supply. Social services agencies work with the displaced, attend to psychosocial needs, and ensure that special needs populations such as the older adults, children, and individuals with disabilities receive the care required. Home nursing associations are often integrated into the emergency response plan to assist individuals with chronic diseases or special nursing needs. The health department is responsible, in most jurisdictions, for coordinating the efforts of the above-mentioned agencies on behalf of the public's health. However, the health department is only one actor in the overall emergency response, which is usually coordinated by a public safety agency such as an emergency management agency, a sheriff's office, or a fire department.

When the resources of the local jurisdiction are insufficient to meet the needs resulting from the disaster, local authorities have the option to call for additional help. The coordinating agency can seek help from surrounding jurisdictions (often referred to as mutual aid resources) or can escalate a request to the state or federal level, or both. The call for outside aid is often called "escalate upward." All states have an emergency management agency (EMA), sometimes called an office of emergency preparedness (OEP). It is the responsibility of the EMA, under the authority of the governor's office, to coordinate the efforts of all state resources used during an emergency or disaster. These resources may be expansive and include the state's health department, housing and social services agencies, and public safety agencies (i.e., state police). In disasters of this magnitude, certain federal resources are made available to the states, such as the National Guard, officers of the CDC (i.e., Epidemic Intelligence Service officers), and the U.S. Public Health Service (i.e., the Agency for Toxic Substances and Disease Registry. Local and state emergency management agencies typically convene a command center away from the disaster site whose function is to coordinate the multiorganizational response of representatives of each pertinent response agency. Health departments should plan to participate in the command center activities as a full partner.

Like a local jurisdiction, states also have the ability to escalate upward if the disaster response requires more resources than the state can quickly provide. Officials can escalate to regional mutual aid compacts or to federal resources. States in many regions of the country are forming multistate regional mutual aid compacts, such as that in the lower Mississippi River region, based on the Central United States Earthquake Consortium. These consortia can provide relatively rapid response due to geographic proximity.

Federal Response

The federal government has developed a federal response plan for the coordination of federal resources used in a disaster situation.[40] The lead agency in charge of coordinating the application of the plan is the Federal Emergency Management Agency (FEMA). The plan consists of 12 sections referred to as "Emergency Support Functions" (ESFs).

1. ESF 1: Transportation
2. ESF 2: Communication
3. ESF 3: Public Works and Engineering
4. ESF 4: Firefighting
5. ESF 5: Information and Planning
6. ESF 6: Mass Care
7. ESF 7: Resource Support
8. ESF 8: Health and Medical
9. ESF 9: Urban Search and Rescue
10. ESF 10: Hazardous Materials

11. ESF 11: Food
12. ESF 12: Energy

Although the federal response to the health needs of disaster victims is detailed in "ESF 8: Health and Medical," all other emergency support functions have both a direct and an indirect effect on the public health sector's ability to protect the health and welfare of disaster victims.

The resources covered by the federal response plan are normally accessed by a request from a state's governor or the state's EMA to FEMA, referred to earlier in this chapter as a presidential declaration. FEMA then contacts the agencies that play the lead role for each ESF. A core concept of the federal response plan is that the responding federal resources work at the behest of, and in support of, the local or state jurisdiction that is in charge of managing the disaster response.[40]

In the case of ESF 8: Health and Medical, the lead agency is the OEP. An office in the U.S. Department of Health and Human Services (DHHS), the OEP has departmental responsibility for managing and coordinating federal health, medical, and health-related social services after major emergencies and federally declared disasters. The OEP also directs and manages the interagency National Disaster Medical System (NDMS). The core of ESF 8 is the NDMS, a multi-agency program that also includes the activities of the Department of Defense, the Veterans Affairs Administration, and FEMA. The NDMS has several core functions. The first function, unrelated to domestic disasters, is to repatriate U.S. military casualties to participating U.S. hospitals where an armed conflict results in too many casualties to be adequately managed abroad. The second function, related to domestic disasters, is to provide a program whereby hospitals across the United States agree to care for civilians who have been injured in a disaster and who can't be cared for where they live. These disaster victims are transported to the participating hospitals by the NDMS. Participating hospitals are "federalized" and all charges incurred by disaster victims are paid either by insurance or by the federal government. The third and fourth functions are the result of an NDMS creation: the Disaster Medical Assistance Team (DMAT). DMATs are designed to provide on-site disaster medical assistance (third function) and to transport victims to definitive care (fourth function) while providing medical support for the transported victims. DMATs are formed locally with approximately 30 personnel, including physicians, nurses, paramedics, and logistics officers. Once trained, the team members gather enough supplies to be self-sufficient and are ready to be transported to distant disasters on short notice. These personnel are temporarily "federalized" so that they can provide services outside of their licensing jurisdiction at the level of their licensure or certification credentials without legal ramifications. There is a public health DMAT based in Rockville, Maryland.

The reach of ESF 8 is broader than just the NDMS/DMAT functions. For example, the CDC in Atlanta maintains personnel who can perform rapid needs assessments from a public health perspective. Some of these personnel are stationed at regional offices of DHHS around the country, shortening the time needed for them to respond to a disaster site.

There is also a growing network of federal, state, and local public health and security agencies working together to prepare for and coordinate the health sector response to terrorist acts using biologic, chemical, or nuclear weapons. At the time of this writing, the exact configuration of this emergency response subsystem and its relationship with existing emergency management agencies is still unclear. The OEP and the National Center for Infectious Disease at the CDC are heavily involved in coordinating the health sector participation in this effort.

Voluntary Agencies

Of considerable importance to the successful provision of good public health response to a disaster is ESF 6: Mass Care. The Federal Response Plan makes the ARC the primary agency responsible for this function, which includes sheltering, feeding, emergency first aid, family reunification, and the distribution of emergency relief supplies to disaster victims. The ARC responds first through its local chapters, then state and regional chapters, which may call on national-level ARC resources if necessary.

A vast array of other voluntary agencies participate in disaster response with functions that contribute significantly to public health outcome. Many of these are church affiliated, such as the Salvation Army, Mennonite Central Committee, and Catholic Relief Services. Some are dedicated solely to disaster-related functions, such as the International Critical Incident Stress Foundation; most have more routine public service and emergency functions that are activated according to the needs of a specific disaster.

International Agencies

A vast array of agencies stand ready to respond to requests for international assistance to protect the public's health after disasters. Multinational UN-based organizations include WHO, UNICEF, the UN High Commissioner for Refugees, and the World Food Program. The PAHO (WHO's regional affiliate for the Americas) has a highly organized Office for Emergency Preparedness and Disaster Relief Coordination, which helps coordinate international health sector response in the Americas. Many national governments have an agency that provides unilateral foreign disaster assistance, such as the U.S. State Department's Office of Foreign Disaster Assistance. Numerous voluntary agencies have gained considerable expertise in responding to postdisaster health needs across international borders. Examples include Médecins Sans Frontières, World Vision, Oxfam, and Save the Children.

A Natural Disaster: A Case Study

The following sections detail a realistic scenario of a major earthquake in Memphis, Tennessee. This scenario is based on research provided by FEMA, the Central U.S. Earthquake Consortium, and various Tennessee and Memphis area agencies. The scenario is as realistic as possible, given the two-dimensional format of this publication. The function of the scenario is to help illustrate how the above-described organizations would respond, to detail their responsibilities, and to provide a sense of the timeline that would evolve. Exhibit 1 provides a timeline for the activities that are involved.

Earthquake Hits

Suppose a 7.2 Richter scale earthquake strikes on the New Madrid fault line, with its epicenter some 75 miles north of Memphis. The earthquake hits in the early afternoon on a work day in late January, with snow on the ground and temperatures hovering a little below freezing. Much of the building stock in Memphis is constructed of unreinforced masonry, leading to massive loss of life, loss of 70 percent of hospital capacity, and a virtual total collapse of the local transport and power grids. Private housing is severely damaged, although not as completely as many of the public buildings in the downtown area.

Initial Priorities

In the first two hours after the earthquake, the local EMS and fire services agencies assess the extent of the damage and initiate the process of locating, extricating, and providing emergency medical assistance to victims. The task is overwhelming, with the sheer volume of those in need complicated by the loss of ambulances from the earthquake, the inability to traverse debris-clogged roads, and the loss of viable hospitals to take patients to. EMS immediately request mutual aid from outside agencies. Given the fact that the surrounding jurisdictions are also affected, such aid must come from much further away and be coordinated by state and federal agencies. Federal DMAT and urban search and rescue teams are requested from FEMA and dispatched within hours, but given the distances they must travel and the difficulties of logistics, such teams do not begin arriving until the following afternoon, more than 24 hours later.

Needs Assessment

During the first two-hour time period, the local and state health departments join with their respective emergency management agencies to staff the command center, an integral part of the IMS. A primary function of department personnel is to conduct an immediate needs assessment. Although the health departments dispatch some of their own personnel to the scene to report on visible signs of what the health sector needs will be, the majority of initial information comes from queries of EMS and fire department personnel, for whom initial assessments are a primary responsibility. Health department personnel contact local hospitals by radio for damage reports and information regarding the influx of victims. They also seek information on the viability of the water supply system and the status of preplanned emergency shelters, usually schools. With this information, the health departments conclude that they have a truly catastrophic emergency on their hands, with the probability of many thousands of injured in need of medical care, massive loss of hospital resources, and an almost total loss of piped water. Early reports on emergency shelters reveal heavy destruction, and a cold night is rapidly approaching.

First Attempts To Meet Victims' Needs

During the next four hours (hours two to six), EMS providers find themselves out of supplies, dealing with patient needs as well as they can. Most patients cannot be transported due to road and hospital conditions, meaning that life-supporting care (including shelter and water) must be provided as well as possible at neighborhood collection points. Medics are not trained to deal with definitive care or long-term patient support needs, so improvisation is needed. Surviving private physicians' offices and facilities staffed by voluntary organization members are used. Some health department personnel scramble to consolidate hospital resources in the remaining facilities that are functional. Others work with the local emergency management agency, the ARC, and other voluntary organizations to rapidly open up and staff as many emergency shelters as possible. Other responders work with state and federal authorities to try to acquire emergency supplies of pharmaceuticals and other medical necessities. Health department epidemiologists work with fire service, EMS, and hospital personnel to try to establish a more accurate estimate of the numbers of injured, dead, and

Exhibit 1

Disaster timeline

Disaster Event

	Pre-event Planning	Emergency Response (0–24 hrs)	Emergency Response (24–72 hrs)	Recovery (>72 hrs)
Tasks	Develop Disaster Plan interagency development hazard analysis resource analysis define concept of operations establish chain of command establish mutual aid resources integration of state and federal resources perform plan drills and exercises establish disaster training update and maintain plan establish resource/equipment caches	Activate emergency operations center Establish communications Conduct damage and needs assessment Search, rescue, and extricate Provide field triage, on-site medical care Establish casualty collection points Transport patients to definitive care Activate mass casualty hospital protocols Request mutual aid resources Mitigate occupational hazards Mitigate ongoing threats and hazards, e.g., HAZMATs, sewage	Integrate state and federal resources Continue rescue and extrication Continue health and medical care If applicable, plan and enact a medical evacuation Begin restoration of public works to essential facilities Establish shelter, potable water supplies, and the delivery of food supplies Ensure the safety of water and food Establish means of sanitation/waste disposal, minimize releases Establish disease surveillance Establish CISM services	Continue medical care Monitor public health and medical care Continue monitoring of food, water, and shelter quality and safety Monitor for disease outbreaks Establish vector control Restore public works Provide disaster grants and loans to families and businesses
Organizations	Work with • Emergency Management Agency • City/County Council • Local: Fire, EMS, Police • Social Services • Public Health • Environmental Health • Public Works • Hospitals • Nongovernmental/Private, e.g., Red Cross, RACES	Coordinate with • Emergency Management Agency • City/County Council • Local: Fire, EMS, Police • Social Services • Public Health • Environmental Health • Public Works • Hospitals • Nongovernmental/Private, e.g., Red Cross, RACES	Seek help from • Emergency Management Agency • City/County Council • Local: Fire, EMS, Police • Social Services • Public Health • Environmental Health • Public Works • Hospitals • Nongovernmental/Private, e.g., Red Cross, RACES • State and Federal Resources: –DMATs, DMORTs –FEMA, CDC –Military	Initiate recovery activities with • Emergency Management Agency • City/County Council • Local: Fire, EMS, Police • Social Services • Public Health • Environmental Health • Public Works • Hospitals • Nongovernmental/Private, e.g., Red Cross • State and Federal Resources: DMATs, DMORTs, FEMA, CDC, Military

continues

Exhibit 1

Continued

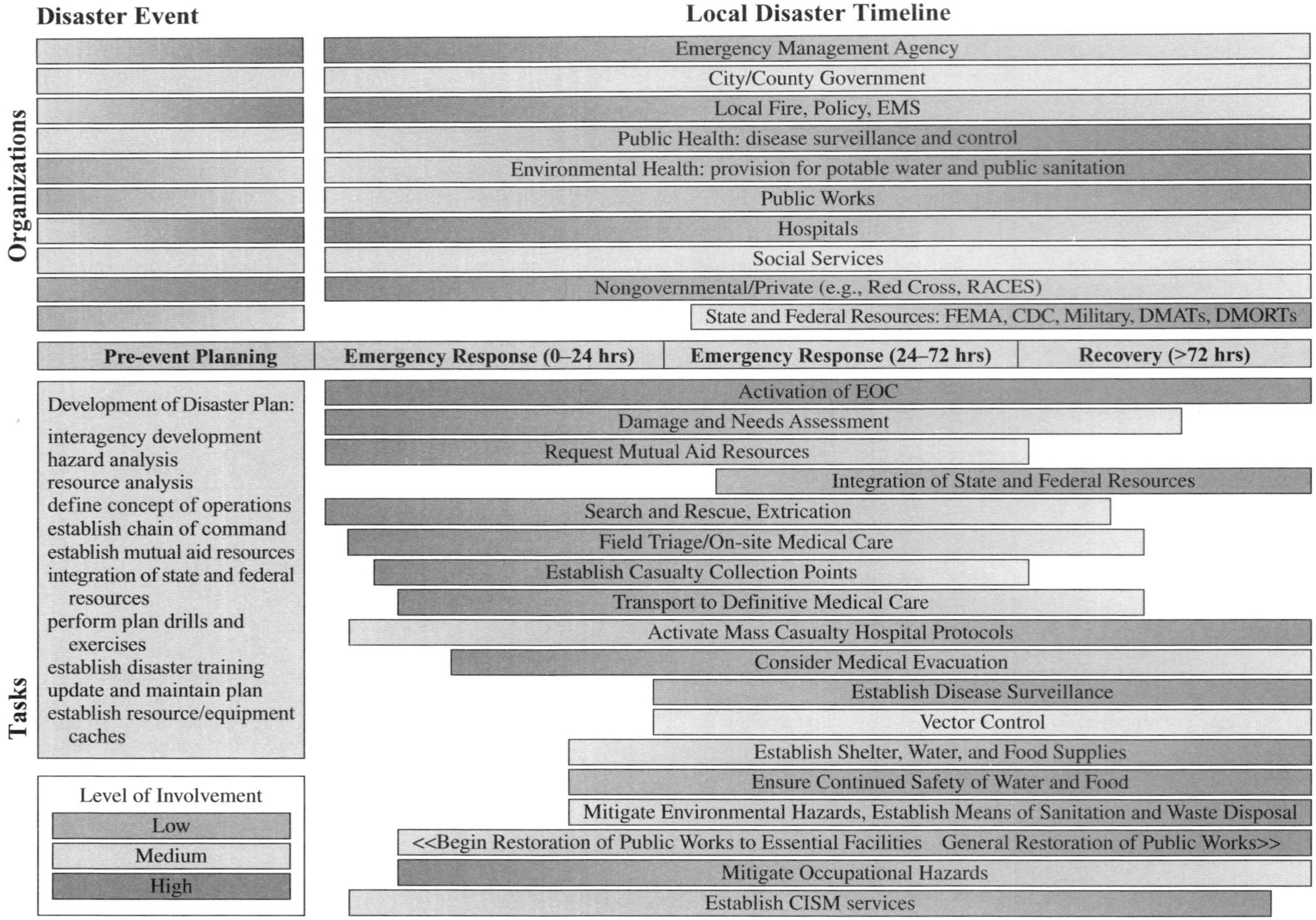

Source: Copyright © 2000, R. Bissell.

those who have other emergency medical needs (e.g., those on oxygen, dialysis, etc.).

Evolving Health Department Actions

As the first 6-hour time period evolves into the first 24, the above roles continue while others come on line. The role that health departments play in ensuring the quality of food, water, and shelter in routine times converts to one of working with multiple organizations to provide those basics, while also working to ensure quality. Emergency shelters can quickly become breeding grounds for infectious disease if proper sanitary measures are not put in place. Likewise, the safety of the emergency water supply becomes an issue of paramount importance. Health departments find themselves working with private and public utilities, housing departments, and a vast collection of private voluntary organizations in order to ensure the provision of basic necessities. Mental health and social services needs also begin to emerge at about this time, adding another layer of agency involvement and increased need for coordination.

Outside Resources Arrive

Approximately 24 hours after the first shaking was felt, many of the outside agencies begin to arrive. This includes such diverse teams as DMATs, urban search and rescue teams, assessment teams from the CDC, specialists from FEMA, emergency morgue workers, and specialists to help assess the need for hazardous materials response teams. At the same time that these broader public health functions are added to the response, the medical community is still trying to provide emergency care for the acutely injured and ill. One of the key tasks of health authorities at this point is to try to find clinicians who can replace or reinforce local clinical personnel who, by this point, are exhausted and often worried about their own families. The NDMS DMATs can help fill this role, but they are too limited in number to meet all of the needs in a catastrophic disaster.

It is the role of public health authorities to begin thinking about returning health care services to normal as soon as possible after a disaster. Although it may seem premature to start thinking about this so soon into the scenario given here, this approach is key in setting priorities during the emergency period.[41] Fire departments and EMS often deal with the complexities of managing a large emergency response by dividing the operation area up into sectors that are functional, geographic, or both. Health departments find it necessary to do the same during the early hours and days of an overwhelming disaster.

Transition from Acute Care to Primary/Preventive Care

Into days three and four, the number of new casualties found who need emergency care diminishes, but the need for acute care continues to overwhelm the restricted capacity of the health care system. Patients present with disaster-related conditions, as well as chronic illness that has become acute in a period of diminished resources. Reestablishment of primary care at this time becomes a high priority and a challenge to health authorities. This is also the period when authorities need to enforce increased vigilance for conditions that are likely to lead to outbreaks of infectious disease. Health authorities seek mutual aid from surrounding or distant jurisdictions in order to provide trained personnel to perform the core functions of case investigation, laboratory confirmation, and remedy.

The Work Continues

Despite the fact that most disasters disappear from the news headlines within a few days of their occurrence, the effects of the event take months, often years, to remedy successfully. By the end of the first week, public health authorities begin the process of planning the health sector's long-term recovery. Although many of the resources needed may not be within the control of the health department, personnel's coordination of diverse resources is crucial to successful recovery. More than ever before, the public will depend on a strong health department to coordinate effectively with the multitude of multidisciplinary agencies and voluntary organizations needed to protect the public's health while the population is struggling to pull their lives back together.

Assessment in Disasters*

Public health, at the local, state, and federal levels, has a major role in assessing and monitoring the nature of disasters and their impacts on communities. These assessments are important managerial tools in preventing morbidity and mortality and in organizing a response.

Assessing the postdisaster situation requires gathering and evaluating information (critical activities in responding to a disaster), recovering from the event, and rehabilitating postdisaster conditions as they are restored to "normalcy." These processes lead to an identification of: (1) the needs of the affected community after a disaster has occurred, (2) appropriate relief goods or services for that community, (3) epidemic levels of disease or injury if indicated, and (4) resources that may be needed by health care services in the disaster zone. From objective and unbiased information produced by such an assessment, informed decisions may be made by health officials or emergency managers to direct response and recovery activities.

**Source:* This material was published in the public domain. No copyright applies.

Measurements of Disasters

Objective measures are used to quantify environmental hazards and human impacts related to natural disasters. To indicate the severity of a disaster event, scales developed by different scientific disciplines such as seismology and meteorology to measure the disaster event are used to describe the hazard from the public health standpoint. For example, the magnitude of an earthquake is indicated by the Richter scale, which provides a measure of the total energy released from the source of the earthquake. The intensity of an earthquake is represented by the measurements on the modified Mercalli scale, which indicates a measure of the degree of damage from a particular location. Similarly, the strength of tornadoes may be measured by the Fujita scale. For hurricanes, the Saffir-Simpson scale is presently used by meteorologists, although recent storms have shown that the scale may need modification to reflect varying amounts of rain, wind, and storm surge.

Measures may also be made of the physical manifestations of a disaster event to indicate the size and severity of that event. For example, the height of a river above flood stage can signal the scope of a flood event. Levels of pollutant aerosols can represent the degree and extent of environmental exposure after uncontrolled forest fires. Levels of pesticides in drinking water or sediment after severe flooding may lead to questions about acute and chronic exposure to toxic chemicals in na-tech events.

Measures of biologic effects, that is, human health effects, indicate resulting impacts on human health and disease. In earthquake events, age-specific injury and death rates may be calculated in cases for whom a direct health outcome is associated with the event. Among displaced persons in shelters where an infectious disease outbreak may occur, laboratory typing of organisms in biologic samples such as blood and urine may indicate exposure to a disease-causing pathogen and confirmation of disease. Similarly, biochemical testing of affected individuals exposed to toxic chemicals via oral, dermal, or inhalation routes demonstrates the presence or absence of an analyte of the chemical compound and the amount of an analyte that may be compared against a reference standard to assess exposure levels. In famine situations, anthropometric measurements, such as height to weight ratios among young children, may indicate the type and degree of malnutrition due to lack of food.

Applied Epidemiology

A systematic approach to assessing postdisaster conditions is based on the principles of epidemiology, the cornerstone of public health science. Epidemiology—derived from the Greek roots *epi* = among, *demos* = people, and *logos* = doctrine—is the study of the occurrence of diseases in human populations.[42] Epidemiology addresses disease occurrence by scientifically measuring characteristics of individuals and the relationships of people to their environments. Classically, epidemiology has been applied to infectious diseases in populations, or "epidemics," and investigators have identified microorganisms that cause diseases, determined infectiousness and immunity among humans, and recommended public health measures to thwart the spread of diseases. In recent decades, however, epidemiologic methods have been applied in many health fields, including environmental health, chronic disease, and injury control.[43]

One recent application of epidemiology is the investigation of the public health and medical consequences of natural disasters. Known as "disaster epidemiology," or "epidemiology in disaster settings," this discipline evolved as scientists realized that the effects of disasters on health were amenable to study by epidemiologic methods.[43] Some of the methods involve a comparison of people who were killed or injured with people who were not in order to learn the ways in which they differed. Epidemiologists identify risk factors with the aim of preventing the occurrence of death.

Applications of epidemiology in disaster settings are conducted for many reasons. Primarily, they are used to describe the health effects of contributing factors, such as demographic characteristics and environmental parameters, and to prevent adverse health effects from occurring in a particular disaster event and in similar events in the future. After 183,000 persons died in a major tropical cyclone that struck coastal Bangladesh, mortality could have been further prevented by effective warnings leading to earlier response actions, access to designated cyclone shelters, and improved preparedness in high-risk communities. In particular, women and children less than 10 years of age were found to be at risk for cyclone-related deaths.[45]

Epidemiologic investigations may also provide informed advice regarding probable health effects. Following the Mt. St. Helens volcanic eruption, a comparison of people who were treated for asthma and bronchitis with healthy matched controls indicated that a history of asthma, and possibly of bronchitis, was a risk factor for contracting respiratory illness. The main exacerbating factor was the elevated level of airborne total suspended particulates, which were greater than 30,000 micrograms per cubic meter after the eruption.[46]

Epidemiologic studies may be used to identify needs in affected communities by rapid needs assessments. Using a list of needs in an affected community, public health authorities or emergency management officials can use these techniques to provide information for emergency planning, provide reliable and accurate information for relief decisions, and ultimately, match resources to needs. A needs assessment conducted two months after Hurricane Georges struck the Dominican Republic indicated the need for food, with special consideration to pregnant and lactating women and their newborns.[47] Finally, managers can employ epidemiologic applications to evaluate the effectiveness of program interventions used to provide relief.

Epidemiologic activities in the impact phase include the following techniques: (1) rapid needs assessment, (2) disease surveillance, and (3) descriptive and analytic investigations. In the immediate aftermath of a disaster, a critical concern of relief authorities is the identification of the needs of an affected community.

- Rapid *needs assessment* or rapid epidemiologic assessment, represents a collection of techniques—epidemiologic, statistical, and anthropological—designed to provide information about an affected community's needs after a disaster.[48] The objective is to obtain timely and objective information or a snapshot of a disaster-stricken community quickly so that immediate actions may be taken for relief activities.
- *Surveillance* refers to an ongoing and systematic collection, analysis, and interpretation of information linked to planning, implementation, and evaluation of public health practice, and closely integrated with the timely dissemination of these data to those who need to know.[49] Often, disease surveillance systems are implemented to signal whether outbreaks of infectious diseases are occurring in the community.
- *Descriptive and analytic investigations* may be undertaken by health authorities in situations where assessment and surveillance raise further questions and hypotheses concerning a health condition in the affected population. These investigations are designed to address questions or test hypotheses so that recommendations can be made for the prevention of any adverse health outcomes related to the disaster event.

The ultimate aim of disaster epidemiology is to determine strategies to prevent or reduce deaths, injuries, or illnesses related to the disaster. Prevention strategies are often grouped into three categories.

1. *Primary prevention*, or prevention of the occurrence of deaths, injuries, or illnesses related to the disaster event (e.g., evacuation of a community in a flood-prone area, sensitizing warning systems for tornadoes and severe storms), is an initial recommendation resulting from descriptive and analytic postdisaster investigations.
2. *Secondary prevention*, or the mitigation of health consequences of disasters (e.g., use of carbon monoxide detectors when operating gasoline-powered generators after loss of electric power after ice storms, employing appropriate occupant behavior in multistory structures during earthquakes, building a "safe room" in dwellings located in tornado-prone areas), may also be instituted when disasters are imminent.
3. *Tertiary prevention*, defined as minimizing the effects of disease and disability among the already ill, is employed in persons with preexisting health conditions and in whom the health effects from a disaster event may exacerbate those health conditions. Examples include appropriate sheltering of persons with respiratory illnesses and those prone to such conditions, particularly the elderly and young children, from haze and smoke originating from forest fires, and sheltering elderly who are prone to heat illnesses during episodes of extreme ambient temperatures.

Emergency Information Systems

Information is critical to any response effort after a disaster has occurred. The need for objective and reliable information is underscored by the nature of the postdisaster setting. First, disasters disrupt normal or existing relationships between people and their physical and social environments. Threats to health may ensue due to changes in preexisting levels of disease, ecologic changes as a result of the disaster, population displacement and movement of survivors leading to overcrowding and situations in which sanitation and hygiene are compromised, disruption of existing services such as public utilities, and disruption of normal public health programs. Moreover, the potential for communicable diseases increases for vectorborne, waterborne, and person-to-person transmission. As such, accurate and reliable information is needed in making decisions about the needs of the affected population for immediate relief efforts, short-term responses, and long-term planning for recovery and reconstruction.

There are several types of information that are collected for decision making, and each type has multiple uses. Deaths are often an initial starting point because they indicate the severity of the disaster event. Using mortality data, managers can assess the magnitude of the disaster event, evaluate the effectiveness of disaster preparedness, evaluate the adequacy of warning systems, and identify high-risk groups where more contingency planning is required. By reviewing information about casualties or the injured, emergency medical personnel and managers of critical care facilities can estimate needs for emergency care, evaluate predisaster planning and preparedness, and evaluate the adequacy of warning systems. Managers can assess information about morbidity, or disease, to estimate the types and volume of immediate medical relief needed, to identify populations at risk for disease, to evaluate the appropriateness of relief activities, and to assess needs for further planning.

In addition to information that helps public health professionals understand the health effects of disasters, information concerning public health resources, particularly from LHDs, is important for emergency information systems. Using these data, officials can estimate the types and volume of supplies, equipment, and services needed for the emergency, can assess needs for further planning, and can evaluate the appropriateness of relief interventions.

In international scenarios, managers can review information about donated goods and the overall relief effort to estimate the types and volume of supplies, equipment, and services needed over time. The goal is to match the appropriateness of the donated goods to the needs and culture of the receiving country, to evaluate the appropriateness of relief activities, and to assess needs for further planning.[50] Wool blankets are not needed in the tropics, and the donation of outdated medication presents the unwanted problem of disposal on a community that is already struggling with enough problems. One example of an information management system is SUMA (supply management program), which was developed by the PAHO and successfully applied in past disasters in Latin America. This computer-based system provides a mechanism for sorting, classifying, and preparing an inventory of relief supplies sent to a disaster-stricken country.[51]

Finally, information may be compiled for hazards, specific events related to those hazards, and health outcomes associated with those hazards. These emergency information systems monitor health events, diseases, injuries, hazards, exposures, and risk factors related to a designated event. An early warning system may forecast the occurrence of a disaster event by monitoring conditions that are likely to signal the event. An example is the Famine Early Warning System that was established by the U.S. Agency for International Development (USAID) to monitor climate and meteorology, availability of food in the market, and morbidity related to nutrition in order to predict the occurrence of famine in undeveloped countries.[52]

Surveillance

Public health surveillance is the

> ongoing and systematic collection, analysis, and interpretation of health data used for planning, implementing, and evaluating public health interventions and programs, closely integrated with the timely dissemination of these data to those who need to know. Surveillance data are used both to determine the need for public health action and to assess the effectiveness of programs. The final link of the surveillance chain is the application of these data to prevention and control. A surveillance system includes a functional capacity for data collection, analysis, and dissemination linked to public health programs.[49(p.164)]

In the postdisaster setting, surveillance provides information that can serve as the basis for action during the immediate disaster and also for planning of future activities.

Postdisaster surveillance is conducted by health authorities primarily to monitor health events. By instituting a surveillance system, one can detect sudden changes in disease occurrence, follow long-term trends of specific diseases, identify changes in agents and host factors for the diseases of interest, and detect changes in health practices for treating relevant diseases. Surveillance also provides tools for the public health practitioner in investigation and control, planning, generating hypotheses, stimulating research, testing hypotheses, and documenting disease activity.[53]

Surveillance is conducted after disasters primarily to detect any illnesses or injuries in the affected population. Information from the surveillance system is used to provide information for decision making by public health authorities. For example, measles vaccination campaigns may be launched in shelters concurrent with normal vaccination programs, with information from the surveillance indicating only sporadic cases. Surveillance is also conducted to investigate rumors, such as the occurrence of infectious disease, which commonly arise in the aftermath of a disaster event. Surveillance data can signal whether an outbreak has actually occurred. If unusual increases of disease are observed, public health workers may be deployed to investigate in order to determine the veracity of the reports and confirm diagnosis. Finally, surveillance is also conducted to monitor the effectiveness of response activities. For example, cases of acute diarrheal disease would be expected to decline with the use and implementation of water treatment interventions. A surveillance system that monitors diarrheal disease where water treatment has been implemented could indicate, as evidenced by rates of diarrheal disease, whether intervention was effective when compared to similar rates from areas without the intervention.[54]

Surveillance systems are usually one of three types: (1) hazard, (2) exposure, and (3) outcome. A *hazard* surveillance is, by definition, an assessment of the occurrence of or distribution of levels of hazards and the secular trends in levels of hazards (e.g., toxic chemical agents, physical agents, biomechanical stressors, as well as biologic agents) responsible for disease and injury. Although no strict methodology exists, a starting point for the surveillance may be to determine the parameters that affect the occurrence, quantity, and distribution of the agents and plot these through time. Alternatively, one could adapt existing information used for hazard surveillance, such as registries of use of toxic substances in compliance activities. An example of the application of postdisaster hazard surveillance is the use of a report of daily variations in respirable particulate matter (i.e., particles with a mass median aerodynamic diameter of ≤10 microns) after wildland fires. Thresholds can be established whereby people who are susceptible to pulmonary disease can be guided to take precautionary measures when the particles reach a certain size.

Surveillance may also be based on *exposure,* which by definition is a characteristic of interest, also known as a risk factor variable, predictor variable, independent variable, or putative causal factor. In disaster settings, exposure may be based on physical or environmental properties of the disaster event, such as "ash fall" after volcanic activity or pesticide-contaminated soil unearthed by flood water.[55] An example of postdisaster exposure surveillance is a report of daily activities, including time of exposure, of outdoor workers who are exposed to "ash fall" after a volcanic eruption.

Surveillance is more commonly based on a health *outcome,* defined as a health event of interest, usually illness, injury, or death. Outcome variables are also known as the response variable, dependent variable, or effect variable. An example of postdisaster outcome surveillance is the Health Impact Surveillance System (HISS) used by the ARC and the CDC. Using HISS, the ARC records mortality and morbidity statistics during disaster events where they are involved.[56]

Other types of surveillance systems may be based on the characteristics and objectives for establishing those particular systems. Decisions need to be made about using existing or temporary systems, hospital-based or community-based systems, and active or passive systems. When deciding to use existing systems rather than establishing temporary data collection systems, managers should consider whether existing systems, such as those for notifiable diseases, would provide adequate and timely information in the immediate aftermath of a disaster. If not, managers can set up temporary systems for the duration of the emergency period, or for the phase in which the information is desired. For hospital-based data collection versus community-based collection, one may consider whether hospital-based data would provide an accurate representation of morbidity related to the disaster. If not, data collection should be extended to include information obtained from mobile care sites or clinics. Given that resources may be finite, monitoring only at sentinel sites may be more appropriate than using a comprehensive "all-sites" approach. The critical issue is whether selected sites will provide a reasonable representation of the health outcomes being monitored. Finally, for active versus passive systems, one may decide that active solicitation of information may provide timely and appropriate information on health effects of a disaster event, in contrast to a passive surveillance system that collects data on similar health effects on a routine basis. Because of the need for information for rapid response and the myriad of health outcomes that may specifically result from a particular disaster event, active surveillance systems tend to fit more of the needs of health authorities in disaster situations.

The importance of public health surveillance may be assessed by performing the following steps:

- Determine the public health importance of monitoring selected morbidity and disaster-related mortality.
- Assess the availability of a public health response based on the data collected.
- Determine any economic impacts on the part of the institutions that will be participating in the system.
- Determine the level of public health concern for the system currently in place.

In establishing a surveillance system, the outcomes of potential importance are first determined (i.e., selected diseases, injuries, and causes of death that are important to monitor after a specific disaster event). Diseases that were endemic in the affected area prior to the disaster event should be included in the system because these would be expected to rise with increased population density, displacement, interrupted normal public health programs, and compromised sanitation and hygiene.

Case definitions for selected health outcomes should be formulated to ensure uniformity of selection in the surveillance system. A case is a unit of observation in the surveillance system with the health condition of interest. Case definitions are criteria for deciding whether a person has a particular disease or health-related condition. These definitions are standardized and are used for investigations and for comparing potential cases. The criteria are applied to individuals under investigation consistently and without bias. Three criteria are commonly used to define the cases: (1) clinical criteria, which are clinical signs and symptoms of disease; (2) laboratory criteria, which are confirmatory tests for disease; and (3) epidemiologic criteria, which place limits on person, place, and time for the development of disease. Once the criteria have been established, cases may be classified into categories: (1) confirmed, (2) probable, (3) suspect, or (4) not a case, defined as failure to fulfill criteria for confirmed, probable, possible, or suspect case. Exhibit 2 lists examples of a decision tree for case criteria.

Exhibit 2

Examples of criteria for case definitions

Coccidioidomycosis after the Northridge earthquake

Confirmed case: onset of signs and symptoms consistent with acute coccidioidomycosis from January 24, 1994, until March 15, 1994, plus laboratory confirmation

Probable case: acute onset of at least four of the following features: fever, chills, cough, pleural pain, erythema nodosum, arthralgias/myalgias, same outbreak period

Possible case: acute onset of at least two of the four features, plus medical diagnosis

Suspect case: unexplained

Not a case: failure to fulfill criteria for the above

Flash flood–related deaths in Puerto Rico

Confirmed case: death that occurred as a direct result of the impact of the floods on January 5 or 6, 1992, and identified by the medical examiner's office

Probable case: death that occurred as a direct result of the impact of the floods on January 7, 1992 (e.g., cause of death would be drowning)

Possible case: death that occurred as an indirect result of the impact of the floods on January 5 or 6 (e.g., cause of death would be myocardial infarction)

Suspect case: unexplained

Not a case: failure to fulfill criteria for the above

Source: Data from (case 1) E. Schneider et al., A Coccidioidomycosis Outbreak Following the Northridge, California Earthquake, *Journal of the American Medical Association,* Vol. 277, pp. 904–908, © 1997, American Medical Association; and (case 2) C. Staes et al., Deaths Due to Flash Floods in Puerto Rico, January 1992: Implications for Prevention, *International Journal of Epidemiology,* Vol. 23, pp. 968–975, © 1994.

Once case definitions have been established and the information for the surveillance period collected, it is important to identify data for comparison, usually from the same time period of a prior year or of the same period extending several years back, when a similar disaster event did not occur. Information from the comparison group provides a reference against which one can determine whether unusual trends or patterns are occurring in the surveillance period.

A successfully implemented surveillance system facilitates the dissemination of information. Proper dissemination would include reports in a form and with content that would alert policy and decision makers, prevention program managers, the media, and the public about information that should be linked to public health action.

Data Collection

Accurate and reliable information is needed for responding to a disaster event and in planning relief and recovery activities. Such information originates from a variety of sources, including predisaster institutions and units created specifically to provide immediate response following a disaster.

Historical information of a disaster event provides a background of the hazards, risks, and vulnerabilities of a particular area. This gives the decision maker an idea about the severity of the occurrence of a disaster event. Officials may use this information for planning disaster preparedness programs, response activities, and evacuation plans. Usually, this information is available from the local civil defense office, geologic institutions, or ministries related to natural resources and the environment. Examples of background information include hazard mapping, microzonation (spatial assessment of risk), frequency and magnitude of geophysical phenomena, and vulnerability assessment. Historical information may be used by emergency managers as a reference against which to compare phenomena exhibited by the disaster event of interest.

During the relief phase, the following data provide useful information for emergency managers and public health officials to gauge appropriate relief efforts:

- demographic characteristics of the affected area and surrounding vicinities
- casualty assessment, including deaths, injuries, and selected illnesses
- assessment of the needs of the displaced population
- coordination of volunteer assistance
- management of facilities
- storage and distribution of relief materials
- communication systems
- transportation systems
- public information and rumor control
- registration inquiry services
- traffic and crowd control

Data for such information may be extracted from a variety of sources, including: (1) existing data sets (e.g., census and national health information systems); (2) hospitals and clinics (e.g., emergency department and hospital records); (3) private providers of health care (e.g., patient records); (4) temporary shelters (e.g., daily shelter census, logs at medical facility in shelter); (5) first responder logs, such as DMAT patient logs; (6) and mobile health clinics, such as those run by the military, nongovernmental organizations (NGOs), and volunteer medical groups (e.g., patient logs, records of prescription medications dispensed).

Population-based sampling techniques, when possible, should be employed if surveys are to be conducted in affected communities. The selection of an appropriate method depends on the objectives of a collection system and the existence of a sampling frame. For instance, if all of the households in an affected area are identified and mapped prior to a disaster event, a simple random sample may be appropriate for a community-based needs assessment. If a sampling frame does not already exist, then a cluster design might be more appropriate. Other designs include a systematic or stratified sampling.

Maintaining confidentiality of health records is given utmost consideration in the collection of data about an individual. If personal identifiers such as names, or identifying numbers that may link a record to a name, are recorded on a form, then the official must ensure privacy and confidentiality of the record. If data at the individual level are collected, informed consent of the patient is obtained in most cases, and information is reported in aggregate form.

Disaster Informatics

Disaster informatics is defined as the theoretical and practical aspects of processing and communicating information, based on knowledge and experience derived from processes in medicine and health care in disaster settings.[57] To date, the development of informatics in disaster settings is fragmented and specific to individual response sectors. In public health, basic computerization is gaining worldwide use, particularly in several disaster-prone developing countries. Scientific literature for public health is accessible via CD-ROMS from selected disaster centers worldwide and is also available on databases on the Internet. Surveillance activities are computer based, with EpiInfo the current software of choice for most postdisaster surveillance systems. However, networks for public accessibility have yet to be developed. Disaster informatics, like most health informatics systems, continues to adapt technology of the future, including high-capacity storage devices (CD-ROMs), networks, new user interfaces, programming tools, higher-capacity processors and increased memory, video and computer integration, voice and pen input, incorporation of a global positioning system and analytic tools for rapid analysis, and use of the Internet and Web sites for rapid access and sharing.

Mental Health Considerations in Disasters: Psychosocial Impacts and Public Health

When most people hear the word "disaster," they tend to picture the trail of physical destruction left in a disaster's wake. More often than not, it is images of injured people and collapsed buildings that come to mind. Yet, just as disasters can flatten trees, break bones, and tear houses apart, so too can they profoundly affect individual well-being, family relations, and the fabric of community life. Depending on the specific circumstances, the psychosocial impacts of disasters can range from mild stress reactions all the way to problems such as substance abuse, stigmatization, depression, and posttraumatic stress disorder (PTSD).

From a public health standpoint, it is important to note that the mental health sequelae of a disaster can be quite widespread. Indeed, in terms of morbidity, the social and psychological impacts of a disaster can greatly exceed the direct toll of physical injuries. Furthermore, sometimes these less-visible effects of disasters can be very long lived, affecting the functioning of individuals and communities years after a disaster strikes. Thus, any effort to help restore the health of a community that has suffered a calamity needs to incorporate mental health issues into assistance and recovery efforts. In this regard, public health professionals have a vital role to play in the prevention, assessment, and response to the mental health effects of natural and technological disasters.

Although it is not widely known, public health agencies and public health professionals are heavily involved in addressing the social and psychological impacts of disaster, and attention to these issues represents a core part of the public health profession's response to disaster.[58] In fact, at the federal level, the Public Health Service is a leader in the field of disaster mental health services. The Public Health Service's Emergency Services and Disaster Relief Branch in the Center for Mental Health Services works closely with FEMA and state and local agencies to facilitate the provision of mental health services after presidentially declared disasters. (The Emergency Services and Disaster Relief Branch and the Center for Mental Health Services are part of the Substance Abuse and Mental Health Services Administration.) Numerous other examples of public health involvement with mental health issues can be found at the federal, state, and local levels.

Mental Health Effects of Disaster

Disasters are life-changing experiences. As Myers wrote, "no one who sees a disaster is untouched by it."[59(p.1)] Similarly, Ursano et al. noted that "no one goes through profound life events unchanged."[60(p.5)] Of course, human beings and human societies are often remarkably resilient, and it is important to remember that the challenge of dealing with a disaster can produce positive responses in individuals and communities. As Tierney explained: "Research shows that, rather than being dazed and in shock, residents of disaster-stricken areas have been found to be extremely proactive and willing to help one another. Pro-social behavior, rather than anti-social behavior, is the norm. To the greatest extent possible, people respond immediately to the demands of an emergency situation, providing assistance to one another and supporting those who attempt to manage the emergency."[61]

If it is useful to note that prosocial behavior is often seen after disasters. It is also important to recognize that disasters are highly stressful, disruptive experiences for individuals, families, and entire communities. During a disaster, people may experience such stresses as loss of relatives, friends, and associates; personal injury; property loss; witnessing death or mass destruction; or having to handle bodies.[62] Loss of one's home can be an exceedingly difficult and disruptive experience. In a review of the earlier literature and a report on their own research, Gerrity and Steinglass highlighted the central importance that homes have in people's daily lives.[63] Not only do homes provide shelter, but they are also closely linked with people's sense of identity and their feelings of stability, connectedness, and safety. "Because homes have enormous psychosocial and practical importance in the lives of families, the loss of a home as a result of a catastrophic event can have a lasting impact on a family."[63(p.221)] Indeed, every aspect of a family's existence can be affected, from family roles and responsibilities to ties with the community.

More generally, survivors of a disaster may have to deal with a disturbing new sense of vulnerability. In a disaster, "the fabric of everyday existence is torn away to reveal danger and risk.... Once something of this nature has happened to a person, it is very difficult...to believe that life can ever be the same again."[64(p.1)] Severe traumas like disaster can shatter the basic assumptions people have about themselves and their world.[65]

The period after a disaster can bring additional stresses, such as grieving for lost loved ones, "adjusting to role changes such as widowhood and single-parent status, moving, cleaning and repairing property, and preparing lengthy reports associated with loss."[66(p.133–134)] Overall, experiencing a disaster "is often one of the single most traumatic events a person can endure."[58(p.101)]

People who have gone through a disaster may experience any of a range of emotional, physical, cognitive, and interpersonal effects, and the numbers of people experiencing stress reactions following a major disaster can be large. A list of common stress reactions to disaster is provided in Exhibit 3.

In general, the transient reactions that people experience after a disaster represent a normal response to a highly abnormal situation. As noted earlier, disasters are highly stressful, disruptive experiences. People are exposed to situations that are well outside the bounds of everyday experience, and such situations place extraordinary demands—both physical and emotional—on people. It would be remarkable, then, if individuals who experience such an extreme situation did not exhibit some physiological or emotional response.

As Myers pointed out, in general, these are "normal reactions to an extraordinary and abnormal situation, and are to be expected under the circumstances."[59(p.2)] Stated another way, "the victims of a disaster are normal persons generally capable of functioning effectively. They have been subjected to severe stress and may be showing signs of emotional strain. This transitory disturbance is to be expected and does not necessarily imply mental illness."[67(p.2)]

According to Young et al., "*mild to moderate* stress reactions in the emergency and early post-impact phases of a disaster are highly prevalent. Although stress reactions may seem 'extreme,' and cause distress, they generally do not become chronic problems."[62(p.15)] As a general rule, a majority of individuals who are exposed to a disaster do not suffer prolonged psychological illnesses.[60]

At the same time, this does not in any sense mean that common stress reactions can or should be ignored in the planning and implementation of a comprehensive public health and human service response to a disaster. On the contrary, programs and services aimed at providing "information about normal reactions, education about ways to handle them, and early attention to symptoms" represent an important opportunity for health and human services agencies to help "speed recovery and prevent long-term problems."[68(p.74)]

Although stress reactions can affect large numbers of people, most stress reactions after disaster tend to be transient. However, a portion of the population touched by a disaster may suffer more serious, persistent effects.

> Research shows that mental health problems can result from exposure to natural and technological disasters. These psychological problems include post-traumatic stress disorder (PTSD), depression, alcohol abuse, anxiety, and somatization. Other kinds of problems, including physical illness; domestic violence; and more general symptoms of distress, daily functioning, and physiological reactivity, have also been documented."[58(p.102)]

PTSD

Because PTSD has been the focus of considerable attention in recent years, it is important for public health professionals who may be involved in disaster needs assessment and response to be familiar with it.

Exhibit 3

Common stress reactions to disaster

Emotional Effects	**Cognitive Effects**
Shock	Impaired concentration
Anger	Impaired decision-making ability
Despair	Memory impairment
Emotional numbing	Disbelief
Terror	Confusion
Guilt	Distortion
Grief or sadness	Decreased self-esteem
Irritability	Decreased self-efficacy
Helplessness	Self-blame
Loss of pleasure derived from regular activities	Intrusive thoughts and memories
Dissociation (e.g., perceptual experience seems "dreamlike," "tunnel vision," "spacey," or on "automatic pilot")	Worry
Physical Effects	**Interpersonal Effects**
Fatigue	Alienation
Insomnia	Social withdrawal
Sleep disturbance	Increased conflict within relationships
Hyperarousal	Vocational impairment
Somatic complaints	School impairment
Impaired immune response	
Headaches	
Gastrointestinal problems	
Decreased appetite	
Decreased libido	
Startle response	

Source: Reprinted from B.H. Young et al., *Disaster Mental Health Services: A Guidebook for Clinicians and Administrators,* 1998, National Center for PTSD.

Traumatic events such as disasters are generally "dangerous, overwhelming and sudden."[69(p.41)] They "have high intensity, are unexpected, infrequent, and vary in duration from acute to chronic."[60(p.5)] In the aftermath of stressful events that are "both extreme and outside of the realm of everyday experiences," some individuals may experience a prolonged stress response known as PTSD.[70(p.29)] Unlike the transient stress reactions so often seen among disaster survivors, PTSD is associated with much greater levels of impairment and dysfunction.[62]

PTSD usually appears in the first few months after a trauma has been experienced. However, this is not always the case. Indeed, sometimes the disorder may not appear until years have passed. Likewise, PTSD's duration can vary, with symptoms diminishing and disappearing over time in some people and persisting for many years in others. It should also be noted that PTSD frequently occurs with—or leads to—other psychiatric illness, such as depression. This is known as comorbidity.[71,72]

For a diagnosis of PTSD to be made, several criteria have to be met. First, there is the nature of the traumatic event and the response it evokes: "the person experienced, witnessed, or [has] been confronted with an event or events that involved actual or threatened death or serious injury, or a threat to the physical integrity of self or others...[and] the person's response involved intense fear, helplessness or horror."[73(p.427–428)] Second, the traumatic event is persistently *reexperienced* (e.g., recurrent distressing dreams, feeling as though the event were happening again). Third, the person persistently avoids anything that reminds him or her of the traumatic event (*avoidance*) and experiences a numbing of general responsiveness. This could involve such things as avoiding activities, places, or people that arouse recollections of the trauma, a diminished interest in activities, detachment from others, and a restricted range of affect. Fourth, the person experiences persistent symptoms of *increased arousal* after the traumatic event. Examples include sleep disturbances, irritability, difficulty concentrating, and exaggerated startle response. In addition, for a diagnosis of PTSD to be made, the duration of the disturbance must exceed one month. Finally, the disturbance must cause "clinically significant distress or impairment in social, occupational, or other important areas of functioning."[73(p.429)]

In a comprehensive review of the international literature on the epidemiology of PTSD, DeGirolamo and McFarlane reported that 16 studies assessing the prevalence of PTSD after disasters have been conducted.[74] Nine of the studies were carried out in the United States and six were carried out in other countries. In studies of natural disasters (including floods, tornadoes, earthquakes, volcanic eruptions), the PTSD prevalence rates ranged from a low of 2 percent (Mt. St. Helens) to a high of 59 percent. In studies of technological disasters, the PTSD prevalence rates ranged from a low of 5 percent to a high of 80 percent.

Although much is known about factors associated with the development of PTSD, and about factors that may reduce the likelihood of developing PTSD, the picture is far from complete. One key factor that researchers have identified is the nature of the trauma that the person experiences. "One of the best predictors of psychiatric illness after a traumatic event," wrote Ursano, Fullerton, and McCaughey, "is the severity of the trauma."[60(p.9)] The greatest risk of PTSD is in persons "exposed to life threat and perhaps, in those exposed to terror, horror, and the grotesque."[75(p.9)] According to Young et al., disaster-related variables associated with long-term adjustment problems include mass casualties, mass destruction, death of a loved one, residential relocation, and toxic contamination.[62] There is evidence that some pretrauma factors have an effect as well. Among the various pretrauma risk factors that have been identified in recent research is a history of prior exposure to trauma.

As might be expected, what happens in a disaster survivor's life after the trauma also appears to affect the risk of developing PTSD.[76] For example, it appears that in many situations, social support may play a role as a protective factor. Armed with this knowledge, and guided by an understanding of current research on PTSD, public health planners and practitioners can work to restore damaged community networks as part of a comprehensive prevention effort.

It is also important to remember that although PTSD is usually associated with primary exposure to trauma, people who have not actually experienced a disaster themselves can still develop PTSD and related symptoms. A study of the spouses/significant others (SSOs) of disaster workers after a major airline crash found that the SSOs "showed moderate levels of posttraumatic distress" even though they had not been direct victims of the crash and had not been exposed to the disaster site.[77] Among other steps, the researchers recommend involving SSOs in debriefing and education programs.[77]

In recent years, researchers have focused increasing attention on ethnocultural issues related to PTSD.[78] A number of studies of disasters in the United States have found differing rates of PTSD or other disaster-related impairment in groups of different race or ethnicity.[79] Because of these and other findings, and because "most research and clinical experience validating PTSD as a diagnostic category was carried out in Western industrialized nations," researchers now recognize "the need for culturally sensitive assessment techniques and the need to identify other posttraumatic expressions of distress...that may be particularly pertinent to non-Western individuals."[78(p.536),80(p.12),81] At the same time, the authors of a comprehensive examination of the ethnocultural aspects of PTSD recently concluded that the PTSD construct continues to have a universal dimension that makes it applicable across cultures. "There are substantive reasons to believe that the experience of trauma has similar biopsychosocial consequences in spite of the fact that different cultural traditions may define and experience reality, personhood, and trauma in different ways."[78(p.538)]

Although PTSD has been the subject of considerable research in recent years, it should be pointed out that there are also other serious problems that can develop after a disaster. Acute stress disorder (ASD) is a relatively new diagnostic category that was added to the *DSM-IV Diagnostic and Statistical Manual of Mental Health Disorders.* ASD is "characterized by posttraumatic stress symptoms lasting at least 2 days but not longer than 1 month post-trauma."[75(p.7)] In addition, "major depression, generalized anxiety disorder, and substance abuse are also well documented after exposure to traumas and disasters."[60(p.8)]

Social Impacts of Disaster

In addition to having the potential to produce PTSD, ASD, depression, and other psychological effects, it is important to bear in mind that disasters can also profoundly affect the *social* health of communities. This was dramatically illustrated in Erikson's study of the Buffalo Creek disaster.[82] The disaster occurred in West Virginia in 1972, when the collapse of a makeshift dam used by a coal mining company sent millions of gallons of waste and debris-filled flood waters roaring into a mountain hollow known as Buffalo Creek. The Appalachian mountain community was devastated: 125 people were killed, many others were injured, hundreds of homes and other buildings were wrecked, and thousands of people were displaced. Survivors, many of whom had witnessed dead and dismembered bodies, suffered a wide array of impacts including nightmares, numbing, insomnia, guilt, despair, confusion, depression, and hopelessness.

But in addition to these individual effects, the disaster, plus an ill-conceived relocation effort, effectively destroyed the fabric that held the formerly tight-knit community together. In other words, Erikson noted, the individual trauma produced by the disaster was accompanied by a collective trauma—"a blow to the basic tissues of social life that damages the bonds attaching people together and impairs the prevailing sense of communality."[82(p.154)] With the social support system that people normally depend on no longer available, recovery from individual trauma, argued Erikson, becomes difficult. Thus, postdisaster public health and human services assistance efforts need to focus not only on service delivery to affected individuals and families, but also on restoring support networks and the health of the community as a whole.

Long-Lasting Mental Health Impacts

The extent to which disasters cause serious, long-lasting mental health impacts is still a matter of some disagreement in the research community. "Studies of the victims of disasters show mixed reactions," Hartsough and Myers pointed out.[68(p.4)] "In some disasters, victims seem to fare well without long-lasting problems. In other disasters, they suffer major mental health problems both immediately and for several years after the disaster."[68(p.4)]

Erikson's sociological case study clearly falls into the "significant impacts" category, as does a long-term follow-up study of Buffalo Creek survivors that was carried out by Green and other researchers.[83,84] In that study, the researchers returned to Buffalo Creek in 1986 to conduct multifaceted diagnostic interviews with survivors. What they found was striking: even though 14 years had passed since the West Virginia disaster, the Buffalo Creek survivors still showed significantly higher rates of major depression, general anxiety, and lifetime PTSD as compared to the nonexposed group.

Studies of other disasters, though, have come to different conclusions concerning long-term mental health effects after disaster. Taylor's study of the Xenia, Ohio tornado is a case in point.[85] On April 3–4, 1974, at least 148 tornadoes hit various parts of the country in what was to be the worst outbreak of tornadoes in U.S. history. The most severely hit area was the city of Xenia, Ohio, where 33 people were killed and between 1,000–2,000 people were injured.

Employing both subjective and objective data, Taylor reported finding that although people did experience various symptoms of emotional distress, there was "an extremely low rate, if any at all, of mental illness as a consequence of the tornado."[85(p.273)] Indeed, "a large percentage of the people reported extremely positive psychological reactions to the disaster event. For example, 84 percent of the population asserted that their tornado experiences had shown them they could handle crises better than they once thought they could, and 69 percent responded that they felt they had met a great challenge and were better off for having met it."[85(p.274)]

What accounts for the dramatic difference between studies of Buffalo Creek and the Xenia study? One factor may be that whereas Buffalo Creek's tight-knit community network was for all intents and purposes obliterated by the flood, most of Xenia's extended support networks remained intact despite the damage caused by the tornado. More generally, when one considers the highly complex nature of disaster situations, the enormous variations that can exist between communities and disaster agents, the differences that exist between disciplines in terms of orientation and approach, and the fact that even the definition of the word "disaster" itself is hotly debated, perhaps it is not surprising that divergent findings have been arrived at by researchers studying different disasters.[86] Clearly, though, there is still much that is not yet fully understood concerning disaster impacts—psychosocial risk and protective factors and the effects of various actions and interventions. Rigorous public health research on these and related topics, therefore, will be critically important in the coming years.

Natural Disasters and Technological Disasters

In recent years, there has been considerable discussion in the disaster research community regarding the similarities and differences between natural and manmade disasters. In practice, of course, the line between the two is not always as clear cut as one might think. If flood waters come into contact with toxic chemicals and spread them around a community, is the disaster natural or manmade? Likewise, if increases in population cause a city to expand into flood prone areas, is the disaster that later results natural or manmade?

To the degree that natural and manmade disasters can be compared, the two, suggest Green and Solomon, "are probably more alike than different."[87(p.164)] Among the things they have in common are "the immediate threat and danger and the potential for ongoing disruption."[87(p.164)] At the same time, however, researchers have pointed to a key difference between natural and manmade disasters: the issue of control. "Manmade and natural disasters differ," wrote Ursano et al., "in the degree to which they are felt to be preventable and controllable."[88(p.xv)]

Natural disasters tend to be seen as part of the order of things, "as acts of God or caprices of nature."[89(p.142)] Such calamities are, to some extent, expected, "since we do not have, and do not expect to have, control over nature."[87(p.164)] On the other hand, manmade disasters are at least in principle preventable.[89] One expects to "be able to control technology, and thus it may be more of a blow to suffer a technological catastrophe (a loss of control), since, by definition, it could have been prevented."[87(p.164)] Thus, the issues of blame and responsibility are central in the aftermath of manmade disasters, and such disasters can produce much higher levels of anger and distrust than natural disasters.

Although many researchers accept that there may be some salient differences between natural and technological disasters, the issue of whether such differences translate into different *impacts* on people is still under discussion. Erikson maintained that the human causation associated with technological disasters brings with it additional distress.[89] People who are victimized by technological disasters, he wrote, "feel a special measure of distress when they come to think that their affliction was caused by other human beings."[89(p.129)] Weisaeth also suggested that technological disasters have a somewhat more severe psychosocial impact.[90] "Technological disasters generally cause more severe mental health problems than natural disasters when they are roughly the same magnitude."[90(p.100)] Similarly, Kliman et al. wrote that "it is harder to achieve psychological resolution and mastery of the losses incurred in human-made disaster than in natural disaster."[91(p.277)]

On the other hand, DeGirolamo and McFarlane noted that two reviews of studies on natural and technological disaster came to different conclusions about whether one type has more severe psychosocial effects than the other.[74] They suggest that the jury is still out on the issue. The "present literature review does not allow any firm conclusion on this point."[74(p.58)]

Psychosocial Impacts, Public Health, and the Challenge of Toxic Disasters

Among the most important new kinds of disaster facing public health professionals and the community as a whole are those involving hazardous materials. As the use of chemicals and radioactive materials has dramatically increased over the past 50 years, so too has the possibility of accidental release and exposure. Unfortunately, when the risks involved in the use of hazardous materials have been coupled with factors such as deficient regulation, insufficient safety and health safeguards, and inadequate emergency preparedness, the result has been serious environmental accidents.[92–94]

Chernobyl and Bhopal are probably the best known examples of these "disasters of environmental poisoning."[64] The 1986 Chernobyl nuclear accident killed 31 people, resulted in the evacuation and resettlement of several hundred thousand people, spread contaminants over a huge geographic area, and has been linked to a dramatic rise in childhood thyroid cancer.[95–97] The 1984 Bhopal chemical disaster in India killed an estimated 3,500 people and injured several hundred thousand others.[98] But in addition to Chernobyl and Bhopal, a host of less well-known chemical and radiologic accidents have taken place across the globe, ranging from relatively small releases to large-scale contamination episodes. In an increasingly complex and interconnected world, no community is immune from the threat of such accidents. Even communities that are far from industrial production or storage facilities can still be at risk from the transport of hazardous materials.

For several reasons, disasters that involve environmental poisoning present new challenges for communities, emergency planners and managers, policy makers, and public health and human service professionals.

- *community conflict:* Typically, after most disasters, people have a tendency to pull together and support one another. As Fritz explained: "The widespread sharing of danger, loss, and deprivation produces an intimate, primarily group solidarity among the survivors which overcomes social isolation, provides a channel for intimate communication and expression, and provides a major source of physical and emotional support and reassurance."[99(p.63)] But in contrast to this kind of *consensual* adaptation or "therapeutic community," toxic disasters frequently produce what Cuthbertson and Nigg called a *conflictual* adaptation.[100] Because contaminants are usually invisible, there is often great uncertainty as to who may have been exposed and who has been affected. The uneven spread of contaminants means that people who live near each other—even on the same street—can have vastly different experiences of the event. In addition, there can be enormous uncertainty as to the degree of risk involved in the present and in the longer term.[100,101] In the face of such ambiguity and uncertainty, and with high-stakes issues involved (e.g., health effects, responsibility for the accident), different understandings can lead to conflict and division. In such a "dissensus community," neighbors may be bitterly divided and vital support networks may not function.[101,102]
- *social stigma:* Although stigma may sometimes affect other types of disaster situations, the social stigma that follows environmental accidents can be remarkably powerful and pervasive. Residents of affected communities may be seen by others as "tainted" and "people to be avoided."[101,103] For example, following a radiologic accident in Goiania, Brazil, people from the city found themselves the focus of fears and discrimination. As Kasperson and Kasperson noted: "Hotels in other parts of Brazil refused to allow Goiania residents to register. Some airline pilots refused to fly airplanes that had Goiania residents aboard. Cars with Goias license plates were stoned in other parts of Brazil."[104(p.102)]
- *widespread and chronic effects:* Whereas natural disasters like a tornado generally have a low point after which things can be expected to get better, in disasters involving chemicals and radiation, there is no clear low point for those individuals who may have been affected. There is considerable uncertainty regarding the consequences of exposure, and damage (like the contaminants) may be invisible. Furthermore, long-term consequences may take many years to develop. Thus, it is not apparent whether the worst is over or is still yet to come.[105] "In a sense," Baum explained, "this pattern of influence extends the duration of victimization."[106(p.37)] Rather than an event taking place and ending, with a recovery process then commencing, the threat from toxic disasters is seen as a chronic and continuing one. People wonder whether contaminants have entered their bodies, and they worry about the health of their loved ones. Even when an accident is officially declared to be "over," it is, in an important sense, not really over for those who may have been exposed.[89] Studies show that the distress produced by toxic disasters can be quite long lived. Bromet et al. observed elevated levels of distress among mothers of young children long after the Three Mile Island nuclear accident.[107] Likewise, in studies conducted 6½ years after the Chernobyl acci-

dent, Havenaar et al. found consistently higher levels of psychological distress among people in the exposed region as compared to a control region.[108]

As Becker noted, this combination of characteristics—conflict, stigma, uncertainty, and chronic distress—can greatly complicate assistance efforts after toxic disasters.[109] At this point, many questions remain to be answered. What kinds of programs and interventions, for example, can be used most effectively to address the problem of pervasive stigma after contamination episodes? How can community fragmentation and conflict best be avoided? What interventions are appropriate for high-risk groups such as mothers with young children? Clearly, there is a pressing need for additional public health and human service research on the difficult challenges posed by toxic disasters.

Prevention As Priority

Numerous professions and disciplines (e.g., psychology, social work, psychiatry, sociology, emergency management, medicine, counseling, nursing, environmental health science, public policy, etc.) have expertise related to the social and psychosocial impacts of disaster. Working closely with those in allied fields, public health professionals have a vital role to play in developing well-integrated, comprehensive, and effective approaches for assessing and mitigating psychosocial impacts.

As in other public health domains, psychosocial assistance efforts strongly emphasize the principle of *prevention*. The primary objective is to help restore "psychological and social functioning of individuals and the community" and limit "the occurrence and severity of adverse impacts."[62(p.4)] In pursuit of this objective, public health and human service professionals generally employ a multifaceted, multilevel approach aimed at helping individuals, groups, and the community as a whole.

Psychosocial assistance services such as crisis counseling "are primarily directed toward 'normal' people responding normally to an abnormal situation, and to identifying persons who are at risk for severe psychological or social impairment due to the shock of the disaster."[63(p.1)] In this regard, outreach is vital. People generally don't see themselves as needing mental health services after a disaster. Individuals don't usually seek out such services, and they may be ambivalent or even resistant to receiving assistance.[59,62] Health and human services professionals, therefore, "must go out to community sites where survivors are involved in the activities of their daily lives."[59(p.4)] Much of the early assistance will be practical in character, ranging from providing information about how to get insurance benefits or loans to helping people with paperwork. "Some of the most important help may be in simply listening, providing a ready ear, and indicating interest or concern."[110(p.2)] Also of importance is providing people with information about what to expect in a disaster, and how to deal with it.

In thinking about public health strategies for responding to disasters, the rebuilding of support networks is absolutely critical. Figley wrote that "the family, plus the social support system in general, is the single most important resource to emotional recovery from catastrophe."[69(p.40)] Loss of homes, and evacuation and relocation, can badly disrupt social support networks just when people most need them. Therefore, it is vitally important for public health and human services workers to help bolster social support networks.[63,111]

Services Provided after a Disaster

Activities and services provided in the aftermath of disaster need to be tailored to the community being served.[59] This means involving stakeholders, community groups, and others in the development and delivery of services.[112] In addition, special services and assistance may be appropriate for vulnerable parts of the population and groups with special needs. Children, for example, require special attention and programs, as well as age-appropriate informational materials. In addition, because children spend much of their time in the classroom, mental health initiatives for children need to involve teachers and schools.[113–115] For a discussion of postdisaster public mental health interventions for children and adolescents, see Pynoos et al.[116]

Among the other groups with special needs in the aftermath of disaster are people with mental illness/psychiatric disabilities and older people.[117] Older adults may have more limited support networks, mobility impairment or limitation, or illnesses. In addition, disasters can "trigger memories of other traumas, thus adding to an increasing sense of being overwhelmed."[62(p.104)]

Also requiring special attention are disaster workers. (See the ARC series entitled "Coping with Disaster.")[118–120] According to Ursano et al., disaster workers "are often hidden victims of disasters and traumas" because "disaster and rescue workers are repeatedly exposed to mutilated bodies, mass destruction, and life threatening situations while doing physically demanding work which itself creates fatigue, sleep loss, and often risk to one's life. They also experience the stresses of their role as a help provider."[60(p.13)]

Among the prevention techniques employed in the disaster worker community are defusing and debriefing. *Defusings* are short (generally 10–30 minutes), unobtrusive, informal conversations intended to provide support, reassurance, and information.[62] *Debriefings* are a more systematic, structured attempt to help disaster workers make sense of their experiences and manage intense emotions. The Mitchell critical incident stress debriefing (CISD) model and variations of it are used in a wide range of settings.[62] Mitchell and Everly described CISD as "a group meeting or discussion about a distressing critical incident. Based upon core principles of education and crisis intervention, the CISD is intended to mitigate the impact of a critical incident and to assist the personnel in recovering as quickly as possible from the stress associated with the event."[121(p.8),122(p.118)] Despite the widespread use of CISD, and the many reports of its value, there is still no consensus in the research community as to the efficacy of CISD. Various studies to evaluate its effectiveness have come to different conclusions, with some demonstrating a positive effect, others showing no clear benefit, and a small number even suggesting a negative impact.[62] Research is continuing.

Among the numerous other activities and services that are typically provided after a disaster to deal with psychosocial concerns are telephone helplines, information and referral services, literature on the emotional effects of disaster, facilitation of self-help and support groups, crisis counseling, public education through the media, information sessions for community groups, grief support services, and advocacy services. For a more detailed discussion of social and psychological assistance efforts after disaster, see Myers, Young et al., and Raphael and Wilson.[59,62,123]

Public health professionals can also identify resources/assets (citizen groups, associations, publications, specialists at nearby universities, etc.) that exist in the community and that may not yet be linked with mental health assistance efforts.[112,124] In addition, public health professionals can work to build community capacity to address social and psychological impacts.[112,125]

Public health professionals can also work to ensure that disaster and emergency plans adequately consider the social and psychosocial dimension. The need to do so is clear. As Ursano et al. pointed out, "If disaster plans do not consider the psychological effects of trauma, the consequences can overwhelm all available services and resources, exhausting rescue workers as well as victims.... The psychological effects of a disaster, manmade or natural, can quickly overwhelm the medical and social rehabilitation resources if they are not recognized and managed."[60(p.5)] Public health professionals can work with local emergency planning committees and other relevant bodies to incorporate social/psychosocial issues appropriately in disaster plans.

Public Health Research

Finally, there is a pressing need for additional public health research on many issues related to the social and psychosocial aspects of disaster. For example, it will be important to understand the public health implications of the prolonged stress caused by chemical and radiologic contamination. (Epidemiologists and other public health researchers who carry out studies in the field should remember that people may be emotionally affected by what they see and experience, even after the disaster is "over." Just because a researcher may not be called a "disaster worker" doesn't mean that he or she is immune to the emotional effects of major disaster. Appropriate caution needs to be exercised.) In addition, because it is vitally important to understand "what works and what doesn't work," public health professionals can join with other health and human service professionals to conduct rigorous evaluation studies of mental health interventions. For a discussion of other research issues, see Gerrity and Flynn.[58]

In sum, social and psychological impacts are a significant part of the morbidity caused by disaster, making them an important public health issue. Public health professionals have much to contribute in addressing the social and psychological issues connected with disasters. Traditional public health emphases and activities, such as prevention, epidemiology, program development, and evaluation, have an important place in efforts to understand and address the mental health impacts of natural and technological disasters.

Public Health Aspects of Environmental Services During Disasters

This section addresses the environmental issues that require public health intervention during disasters. The section details methods to safeguard the population from disease related to sanitation, personal hygiene, the water supply, diarrheal disease, heating and shelter, and violence. The section concludes with guidelines for environmental surveillance.

Context

A clean environment is the foundation on which healthy populations rely. For example, most of the health benefits (lower crude mortality rate) seen in North America over the past century are due to improvements in the environment. Of the three major killers at the turn of the twentieth century in the United States—(1) influenza and pneumonia, (2) tuberculosis, and (3) gastrointestinal illness—influenza and pneumonia death rates are less than 1/10 of the 1900 rate; the other two are less than 1/1,000th of the 1900 rates.[126] The reductions in these disease and mortality rates occurred primarily before the advent of antibiotics, and came about from improved housing, improved heating and ventilation, improved water supplies, sewage availability, improved food hygiene and refrigeration, and improved food supply (and, in the case of tuberculosis, quarantine/isolation efforts).[127]

However, during a disaster, these "foundations of health" are often lost. The consequences of diminished environmental conditions vary widely from location to location, depending on the diseases present, the susceptibility and habits of the population, and the availability of other redundant protective measures. Diseases that are widespread and have a short transmission cycle and incubation period are the illnesses that arise most readily and rapidly. Respiratory infections and diarrhea are the primary examples. Therefore, the goal of the sanitation or environmental health specialist following a disaster is to replace or repair the existing sanitary barriers as quickly as possible.

Although the environmental actions taken in developed nations during a disaster may seem unrelated to those steps taken during crises in the world's poorest nations, the guiding sanitary principles are, for the most part, the same. In developed nations, the hazards of concern are varied and often include chemical and radioactive hazards. In undeveloped nations, the hazardous material that is usually of primary concern is human feces and the pathogens associated with it. Nonetheless, the task of the environmental health specialist is remarkably similar in these disparate settings.

General Principles

The field of environmental health is based on the concept that certain hazards move through the environment and cause harm to humans. Control measures can be focused on preventing the creation of the hazard, preventing the transport of the hazard, or preventing people from being exposed to the hazard once they encounter it. In the case of malaria control, the three areas of prevention above would correspond to preventing mosquito breeding by draining stagnant water, spraying for mosquitoes to prevent the transport of pathogens, and getting people to use impregnated bednets or insect repellent to diminish exposure opportunities. Whether the subject is diarrhea prevention or toxic waste control, these three types of preventive measures can apply.

As a general premise, no environmental measure functions perfectly 100 percent of the time. In developed countries, this is compensated for by having multiple sanitary barriers between the hazard and a population. For example, in the case of surface water supplies, source waters are protected from pollution, dramatically reducing the pathogen content of water before it reaches the treatment plant. Then, solids are settled out, removing most of the remaining pathogens. After which, water is filtered and chlorinated. If, on a given day, one of these four measures is not functioning, the others will keep the hazard to the public relatively low. Most waterborne outbreaks in developed countries occur when a series of mishaps cause several of the public health barriers to fail. The extent to which a population is free from environmental hazards depends on how aware responsible officials are of the risk and how willing they are to invest in the multiple barriers needed to keep the population's risk low.

A second sanitary principle is that distance aids safety. In general, the more dangerous a substance is and the more volume that exists, the more space that will be allotted to a site. This is because the more distance that exists between a hazard and a population, the more time will generally elapse between any inadvertent release of a hazard and the time when the population is exposed. The word release here means the intentional (e.g., a person defecating in the open) or unintentional (e.g., a break in a pipe conveying a hazardous material) deposition of a potentially hazardous material into the environment. Time allows for more opportunity for the release to be detected, and more opportunity for the population to take measures to protect themselves. Finally, most pollutants degrade or disperse over distance. Therefore, providing space for hazardous material may cut down on human exposure regardless of treatment or containment inadequacies.

Within the context of an emergency situation, where people have been displaced from their homes and may now exist in overcrowded conditions, these general premises of sanitary engineering become problematic. Resources are usually limited, and services must be established at very short notice. This makes the concept of multiple sanitary barriers seem impractical if not absurd. Moreover, displaced people are normally shunted onto the only unclaimed land available, and having "extra" space to separate people and their nearest hazard becomes an impossibility as well. Thus, the practice of environmental health becomes quite crude when applied to displaced populations and refugees. The principal hazard created within these settlements is usually feces. Because its creation is unavoidable, the task of the sanitarian is to minimize fecal transport and to minimize the population's exposure, which in the case of fecally transmitted illnesses means minimizing oral ingestion.

During natural disasters, the task of the environmental health specialist is usually either to protect or to restart the protective barriers that exist, or else to promote changes in behavior that will compensate for the disrupted sanitary barriers. Examples of such messages include orders to boil water, warnings about foods that may have spoiled during electrical outages, or announcements regarding where potable water will be provided. For displaced populations, all basic services usually need to be restarted from scratch. During natural disasters, especially in developed countries, there may be few commonalties between the same types of crises in different locations. Typically, the infrastructure to provide safe water and food is in place; it may simply be inoperative for the moment. Responding quickly and effectively is most often dependent on the local officials' organization and the prepared plans for dealing with crises.

Sanitation

Reviews of epidemiologic studies examining the causes of diarrheal illness in undeveloped countries have shown that the use of latrines or other excreta-containment facilities is more protective than any other environmental measure. Thus, during an emergency, establishing a sanitation system should be one of the first measures undertaken. The appropriate type of facility varies between settings and cultures, although several overriding concepts always apply.

- The purpose of a sanitation system is to contain human excreta at the moment of defecation so that it is not free to spread throughout the environment. Therefore, getting as many people to use the excreta-containment facilities as often as possible is an essential part of all sanitation programs. In some cultures, this may include building separate latrines for men and women or separate latrines for children. In some settings, latrines may be needed in work or gathering areas. Whatever the circumstances of a crisis, if the local workers implementing the sanitation program communicate well with the population being served and understand that their goal is for everyone to use proper facilities all of the time, an appropriate sanitation service will eventually arise.
- People's excreta poses little hazard to themselves. Some researchers have speculated that feces from one's family members is less hazardous than feces from others because families are likely to have common immunologic histories and exchange pathogens on an ongoing basis. Thus, to the extent possible, households should not share latrines or toilets with other households. Because latrine cleaning and mainte-

nance is an unpleasant task in virtually all cultures, having one latrine per household will also increase the likelihood that the facilities will be kept clean. However, the increasing health benefit with increasing coverage needs to be balanced against the time, effort, and expense of building excreta-containment facilities. Populations that are unstable or are expected to be moved within days, such as in complex emergencies in developing countries, are perhaps better served by a communal latrine system. Both UNHCR and UNICEF propose a minimum coverage target of 20 people per latrine, although this level of coverage is rarely achieved in transit and reception centers.

- Mortality and morbidity rates among displaced populations in the first days and weeks of a crisis are often many times higher than rates among the same population once it is stabilized. Thus, providing some sanitation facilities during the first days of a crisis is critical. This means that either latrines of some kind need to be built before the population arrives at a site (which is rare) or defecation fields need to be established. Because defecation fields need to be located away from water sources, not too far from the people who will use them, and in rainy climates downhill from living areas, reserving the proper spaces for defecation fields must be done at the outset of a crisis.
- Young children pose a particular concern for excreta-control programs. This is because children experience a disproportionate amount of diarrhea among population members, thus shedding the most hazardous feces. Also, their defecation habits are particularly difficult to control. Dealing with this problem usually involves two approaches. Educate child-care providers about proper handling of children's feces and the importance of washing their hands after cleaning the child or handling the child's feces. Second, make excreta-disposal facilities that are child-friendly available. Typically, child-friendly latrines are not dark (perhaps even have no walls) and have an opening that is smaller than in an adult latrine.
- Most latrine/toilet options perform the primary task of containing excreta whether they are above-grade barrels, pit latrines, or solar-heated composting toilets. The habits and beliefs of the served population will be the primary determinant in the effectiveness of the structures and materials provided. The process of matching the proper hardware and educational inputs to the beliefs and habits of a population is best done by that population itself. This means that having locals construct and implement sanitation facilities, especially if each household can construct latrines for themselves, is perhaps the most effective way to ensure that facilities will be used and maintained.

Sanitation Options

A brief summary of the characteristics of the most common sanitation options is presented in Table 3.

Personal Hygiene

No area of environmental intervention is more difficult to conduct well than personal hygiene promotion. Whether the issue is poor hand-washing practices among relief workers—which caused diarrhea during the Oklahoma City bombing—or if it is the food reheating habits of Burmese refugees, personal habits can influence a population's well-being regardless of the infrastructure and resources provided. Not only do cultural practices vary between peoples, but different languages often do not have comparable concepts for notions such as privacy or diarrhea. Therefore, as with sanitation, local professionals are best suited to develop and deliver any hygiene education program. Regardless of the setting, several basic premises are universal, specifically, soap provides protection from diarrheal illness independent of any educational program that may accompany it.[128] As people need to be able to clean themselves after defecating, materials for cleansing (paper, sticks) should be made available along with water and soap.

Hand washing, particularly after defecating and before preparing food, has been shown to be protective against fecal–oral illnesses. No studies examining the impact of personal hygiene that were included in a recent review found health benefits associated with education alone, only with documented changes in behavior.[129] Therefore, any efforts to promote hand washing should have a simple monitoring component to ensure that increased hand washing is actually occurring.

Table 3

Sanitation options in disaster response

Characteristics	Defecation fields	Latrines	Flush toilets
Physical description	An area near where people live, reserved for defecating	A pit in the ground covered with a platform; people defecate through a hole in a platform	A basin that is flushed with several liters of water to carry away the wastes through a pipe
Speed of implementation for large populations	Can be established within hours	With an organized program, a communal (shared) system can be established within days	Requires weeks or months depending on the availability of piped water and sewage treatment requirements
Typical cost	<$1 per household	$4–300 per household ($7–30 most typical)	>$50 for pour-flush >$100 for most
Most appropriate setting	Arid climates, abundant space, and a culture used to defecating with little privacy	A population accustomed to using latrines, good soils, and no high water table	Piped water available and plentiful; abundant financial resources
Main public health concerns	People will not use; people will be exposed to excreta while entering or exiting the area	Communal latrine may not be kept clean; people (especially small children) may not use	Water outages from electrical problems or water shortages; flooding can stop treatment

To work, educational messages should be short and focused. An educational campaign with six hygiene messages was promoted by the International Committee of the Red Cross in Tajikistan during a typhoid fever outbreak in 1997. An evaluation of the campaign found that people who received and understood the messages were as likely as those who had not to develop typhoid fever. In this case, only one of the six messages, "Boil your drinking water," had any relationship with the route by which the disease was being transmitted. All messages included in an educational campaign should promote measures known to prevent the specific health threat at hand and should focus on behaviors that are not presently practiced by a significant portion of the population.

Water Supply

Water sources fall into three general categories: rainwater, surface water, and groundwater. In general, *rainwater* collection is not reliable enough to provide water for a large population and is rarely used during complex emergencies. *Surface water* is water that is found in lakes, ponds, streams, and rivers. Surface waters have the advantages of being easy to withdraw and are of predictable reliability and volume. They have the disadvantage of generally being microbiologically unsafe, and thus require treatment. *Groundwater* sources tend to be of higher quality microbiologically, but are relatively difficult to access, and energy is needed to bring water from within the earth's crust up to the surface.

Water quality is usually evaluated based on the presence of some bacterial measure, which indicates the possible presence of feces. Because human feces typically contain tens of millions of bacteria per gram, even minute amounts of feces in water are often detectable via bacterial monitoring. Fecal coliforms are a general category of bacteria that are empirically defined to match the characteristics of bacteria found in the stool of warm-blooded mammals. Finding no fecal coliforms in untreated water is a good indication that there are no fecal–oral bacterial pathogens present, although finding fecal coliforms in water does not prove that the water is dangerous. UNHCR considers water with less than 10 fecal coliforms per 100 ml. to be reasonably safe, whereas water with more than 100 fecal coliforms is considered to be very polluted. Other indicator bacteria, such as *E. coli*, fecal streptococci, or total coliforms, operate on the same premise that absence implies water safety. Contaminated water sources should never be closed until equally convenient facilities become available.

Although water sources may be of differing water quality, in many if not most settings, the handling and storing of water by people will be the main determinant in water safety. Studies have shown that the dipping of water from household storage buckets causes considerable contamination, and that water quality deteriorates over time after the water is initially collected. The best assurance that clean water will stay clean is to add a chlorine residual to the water. This means that in unsanitary settings, or during times of outbreaks, it may be appropriate to chlorinate safe source water. Exhibit 4 provides additional information about surface and ground water.

Water Quantity

In developing countries, epidemiologic evidence indicates that providing people with more water than they currently have is more protective against fecal–oral pathogens than is providing people with cleaner water.[129,130] UNHCR purports that people need at least 15–20 liters of water per person per day (l/p/d) to maintain human health. Although water availability is influenced markedly by the setting where one is working, more water can almost always be obtained with more resources, be they more wells, trucks, or pipes. Because the acquisition of water in arid areas is generally expensive, and the relationship between water quantity and health is somewhat stochastic, there is a tendency to not invest in enough water infrastructure because other demands seem more acute. This makes the documentation of water availability a key component of a public health program during a crisis.

Water consumption should be estimated at least weekly during a crisis. Often, the local utility or NGO providing water to a population collects these figures. Note that water consumption means what people receive, not what the water operators produce. Discrepancies frequently arise between "production" and "consumption" estimates—water can be lost or wasted during pumping and transport, and people may be prevented from getting adequate quantities because they don't have containers to hold water. Therefore, sampling that documents people's use of water (such as household interviews) or the

Exhibit 4

Getting and treating water in a crisis situation

Surface Water

Bucket Collection: Where people collect water directly from water bodies in buckets, the only treatment of surface water that can easily be achieved is chlorination. Water can be chlorinated in the home or by health workers at the point of collection. Ideally, enough chlorine should be added to the bucket so that after 30 minutes, there is still at least 0.5 mg/l free chlorine in the water.

Pipe Distribution: In systems that have many broken distribution pipes or during times of disease outbreaks, attempting to have 0.5 to 1.0 mg/l free chlorine is appropriate. During crises or conflicts, pressure intermittency in pipes allows water to be drawn in through cracks, resulting in cross-contamination responsible for most major waterborne outbreaks. Monitoring of chlorine is recommended to achieve a dose allowing free chlorine throughout the system.

Groundwater

Spring: A location where groundwater flows to the earth's surface of its own accord. To protect the water from contamination, build a spring box, which is a collection basin with an outflow pipe at or below the point where the water comes to the surface.

Wells: To prevent contamination with surface water, the well usually includes a skirt around the opening of the well, or a plate sealing off the surface at the top of the well. Where there is household water contamination or high risk of a waterborne outbreak, water disinfection of wells and springs with chlorine is advisable.

Wells can be of a variety of sizes and shapes, with a variety of pumps or devices to raise the water. Although many reasons relating to siting and construction errors can cause a well to never come into service, wells that operate for a time typically fail because of lack of maintenance and repair capacity. Thus, groups planning to build wells need to budget from the outset for parts and personnel to maintain the projects until local wealth and economic activity can sustain the water system, or until the wells are abandoned.

actual collection of water at watering points is a preferable method of assessing usage than to divide the water produced at a well or a plant by the number of people served. Cholera outbreak investigations have revealed that not owning a bucket puts families at increased risk of illness or death.[131] Thus, not only should the average water consumption be 15 l/p/d or more, but there should not be anyone with very low water consumption (<5 l/p/d) in the population.

During natural disasters in areas with piped water, rapid surveys can quickly determine which areas are lacking in water service. Areas where service is expected to be cut for days or weeks are often vacated, or else water is transported to the area by vehicle. It is not common in the United States or Europe for acute water shortages to result in morbidity or mortality.

Specific Outbreak Control Strategies for Epidemic Diarrheal Diseases

For several specific fecal–oral diseases, different combinations of environmental measures have been shown to be more effective than others. This becomes important when trying to choose the one or two messages to be included in a campaign and when available staff and resources limit the environmental programs that can be undertaken. Exhibit 5 describes control strategies for four major diarrheal diseases.

Exhibit 5

Control strategies for epidemic diarrheal diseases

Cholera: Cholera is perhaps the most waterborne of all diarrheal diseases. Food has also been seen as the main route of transmission in many outbreaks, although foodborne outbreaks are typically less widespread and less rapidly occurring than waterborne outbreaks. Thus, the first task during a cholera outbreak is to make sure that the water people are consuming is chlorinated. In this setting, chlorinated water is considered to be water with a chlorine residual of at least 0.2 mg/l at the moment it is consumed. Where chlorination is not possible, a lemon per liter has been shown to be effective in killing the bacteria that causes cholera (*Vibrio cholerae*), as is boiling water. Because *vibrios* grow well in unrefrigerated foods, efforts to ensure that people have the fuel needed to heat their food adequately is also called for. Adding acidic sauces such as tomato sauce to foods has been shown to be protective against foodborne cholera. Educational efforts should focus on getting people to consume only chlorinated or boiled fluids and eat only hot, cooked foods or peeled fruits and vegetables. Handwashing practices among those who prepare food for others should also receive attention.

Typhoid fever: Typhoid is also a water- and foodborne disease caused by the bacteria *Salmonella typhi*. Ensuring that the water supply is chlorinated is the best assurance against a massive outbreak, as most large outbreaks are waterborne. Many smaller outbreaks are foodborne, with the hands of the food handlers being the primary hazard. Thus, food hygiene efforts should focus on hand washing among food handlers and ensuring that infected people do not prepare food for others. Although most people, once infected, stop passing the bacteria shortly after regaining their health, 10 percent of people will still be shedding three months after the onset of symptoms. Therefore, keeping food vendors with typhoid fever away from work until they are noncommunicable takes considerable effort.

Shigella: Outbreaks of *Shigella Dysentarie* Type I have become quite frequent during periods of civil unrest in recent years. Case fatality rates for this illness can exceed 10 percent. Other forms of dysentery generally follow the same transmission patterns. Because the infective dose of shigella species tends to be low, perhaps less than 100 organisms, hand-to-mouth or person-to-person transmission is more important than with many other waterborne diseases. Several epidemiologic studies have even linked shigella transmission to flies. Strategies for control need to focus on a comprehensive personal hygiene program (soap and plentiful water made available, handwashing promotion), along with water chlorination and food hygiene efforts. Secondary cases within the households of shigellosis patients are common, so outreach programs should focus education efforts on those households where cases occur.

Hepatitis E: Although hepatitis E is fairly uncommon, it disproportionately strikes refugee populations. During major outbreaks, water has been the main route of transmission, although the most common fecal–oral hepatitis, hepatitis A, is transmitted by food and other routes also. This illness is particularly lethal to pregnant women. Thus, control measures should focus on chlorinating water for the entire population and equipping and educating pregnant women about the need for personal and food hygiene.

Heating and Shelter

Although often not thought of as a health issue, heating and shelter have been essential components of disaster responses recently in Europe and the former Soviet Union. Although cold conditions are widely associated with the medical conditions of hypothermia and frostbite, symptoms of malaise and nutritional shortages probably result in more morbidity. Living in cold conditions, even with proper clothing, requires more caloric intake to maintain the same activity level. In general, approximately 1 percent more calories is needed for each degree below 20° C. Thus, someone whose house is 10° C requires 10 percent more food intake to sustain his or her activity level. Rarely does food availability or intake level increase during times of energy hardship. Thus, the metabolic response to cold is for people to slow down. Surveys in Bosnia and Armenia during the early 1990s found that many people were sleeping 18–20 hours per day.

In very cold climates, several things can be done to reduce the hardships associated with cold. High-energy foods such as oil can be made available. Plastic sheeting can be handed out to cover windows and unused doorways. Getting several people or households to share one common heated place can also be useful. In multistory buildings, the temperature in living areas can be dramatically increased by organizing structures so that each floor or apartment heats the same room, causing the heat loss from the floor below to pass into the heated room above. Blankets and sleeping bags can also help people conserve energy during hours of sleep.

In many areas, populations are not used to burning fuels at home as a source of heat. Moreover, during times of crisis, the quality of workmanship and materials may be less than ideal, resulting in either gas leaks or carbon monoxide buildup inside of living areas. Educational messages should warn people about the signs of carbon monoxide poisoning and how to check for gas leaks.

A second area of inexperience has to do with the actual act of burning. Many people are concerned about getting the heat from the fire into the home, and will therefore not build the fire in an insulated stove. At low temperatures (230–300° C), combustion of carbonaceous materials yields carbon monoxide, whereas at higher temperatures (400°+), combustion is generally complete and yields carbon dioxide and approximately twice as much energy. The idea that stove makers should try to keep the heat in around the combustion center is often counterintuitive and requires some education. Likewise, people without a history of burning wood rarely appreciate how important it is to let wood dry for months or years before it is burned. "Green" wood burns cooler (incompletely) because it is laden with water, energy is wasted boiling away the water in the wood, and it is more likely to lead to creosote buildup and chimney fires. Thus, it is very possible that a freshly cut piece of wood will give off less than one-third of the energy it would produce if it were burned after two years of drying.

In warmer climates, sheeting to keep people dry during rainstorms and to provide shade in the daylight can be important for improving the quality of life. Sheeting can allow for the rapid construction of shelter and is often taken by displaced populations when they return home.

Vector Control

Vector control is usually, and perhaps unfortunately, not done during crises. In the United States, mosquito spraying and mosquito monitoring can be a major component of a posthurricane public health program. In developing countries, rat control (particularly in food warehouses), mosquito spraying and eliminating breeding sites, distributing impregnated bednets, dipping cows, spraying for housefly and tsetse flies, setting fly traps, and delousing a population have all been done repeatedly among refugee settings. Usually these measures are taken because of a specific health threat. The most common measures and the most common motivations are as follows:

- Rat control is usually undertaken primarily to limit food and material losses. Rats destroy food and packaging, chew on the insulation of wires, and are generally seen as unsanitary. Thus, many if not most food warehouses will attempt to control rats with poisons, traps, cats, or some combination thereof. Rats can transmit a myriad of diseases such as plague, leptosporosis, and salmonella, although the cost-effectiveness of health improvements through rat control is largely undocumented.
- Mosquito control is often seen as an essential effort where malaria is a major cause of morbidity. Reducing breeding sites is an inexpensive and

safe measure that is often undertaken either formally or informally. Efforts to distribute bednets to Burundian refugees in Tanzania were less than successful according to the International Rescue Committee; in Thailand, similar efforts were favorably evaluated. Spraying for mosquitoes has been done but is often seen as expensive or environmentally unsound.

Mosquito monitoring is widespread in the United States and can be a useful tool following storms and floods for assessing the risks of mosquitoborne illnesses. Some programs trap mosquitoes, whereas others monitor infections in sentinel animals that are placed in locations where they are readily bitten by mosquitoes.

Delousing of refugees (the killing of body lice with chemical applications) is called for when the risks of typhus are perceived to be high and where many people are infected with body lice.

Violence

Violence is becoming a more common problem during the relief phase of a crisis. Although this can be seen as a political or nonhealth issue, recent crises in Kosovo, Bosnia, and Rwanda have seen violence as the major cause of morbidity and mortality—making it THE public health issue. Thus, documenting the time, place, and extent of the violence becomes part of the responsibilities of the public health system.

For the environmental health specialist in developing countries, three facets of violence are particularly important: land mines, intentional water cuts, and protecting people as they obtain and transport water. Land mine risk happens over space. Documenting where mines have gone off and where they have been found and publicizing this information is an important task in keeping a client population safe. The intentional cutting of water supplies to a population, as occurred repeatedly in Bosnia, should be documented and reported to those UN or human rights officials who are most likely to influence the political forces causing the crisis, or to be involved in any tribunals that may occur. Finally, providing people with water in a place and fashion that minimizes their risk is becoming a greater and greater part of water provision services. This may require piping water to populations rather than having them venture into dangerous areas, or may simply mean placing taps under overhangs so that people are not exposed to snipers as they wait in the queue.

It is no longer sufficient to focus on preventing waterborne diseases when designing water supply schemes. The goal should be to prevent all water-related hazards. In Sarajevo during the 1993–94 period, the main hazard associated with the water supply was being shot by snipers while collecting water. Thus, UNICEF and the other NGOs involved in water provision appropriately began providing water to locations that snipers could not view.

Environmental Surveillance

The quantitative monitoring of services is an essential part of an effective environmental health program. The monitoring process allows for an accurate estimate of how conditions are changing over time. More importantly, having a numeric estimate of service levels or service quality often improves the service either by making the monitored workers more conscientious or by adding political impetus. Often, the process of surveying keeps workers in touch with the people being serviced and enables them to notice ancillary issues to the parameters being measured.

Monitoring information should be graphically displayed in a public location. This will increase the awareness of the efforts underway for people in other programs and the client population. Programs for which the level of indicators is favorable will help inspire other programs. Programs that are not meeting their goals may get suggestions, help, or even prodding from others, which may help the effort. Many examples have arisen where NGOs did not quantify water availability for specific populations, and the eventual measurement of insufficient quantities allowed for the acquisition of more resources to alleviate the problem. The monitoring of household levels of free chlorine by the International Federation of the Red Cross (IFRC) in Dushanbe during the latter part of 1997 through 1998 is largely responsible for the improved reliability of chlorination by the water utility and the avoidance of another widespread typhoid outbreak during 1998. When the surveillance started, less than half of the households in Dushanbe had measurable chlorine in their taps. After several months of monitoring and lively exchanges, the water utility managed to maintain a chlorine residual throughout the entire city.

Certain parameters, such as fuel and soap availability, need to be monitored only when the situation dictates. In some settings, such as when people are still in their houses and have electricity, people have all of the fuel they need and monitoring the average hours of electrical service is a more demonstrative indicator of their conditions. There are three parameters that always call for a numeric estimation.

1. *access to excreta disposal facilities:* The number of people per latrine articulates both the relative availability of latrines and the amount of sharing that is occurring.
2. *water consumption:* Estimates can be obtained by 24-hour recall interviews with a representative sample of the population or by monitoring how much water is collected at the various sources and dividing this by the number of people being served. Water consumption is always articulated as liters per person per day.
3. *percentage of people consuming safe water:* The host government or overseeing UN agency usually has a microbiologically based criteria for considering water safe. If none is available, use <10 fecal coliforms per 100 ml. water. Water with any detectable free chlorine residual should be considered safe. The fraction of people who are getting "safe" water at the time of collection should be monitored.*

Crises tend to destroy the sanitary barriers that in times of tranquility help maintain the health of a population. In natural disasters, the general goal is to reestablish the sanitary barriers as quickly as possible. This requires planning and organization before the crisis occurs. Displaced populations always require food, water, and some type of sanitation services. Establishing these services requires a predictable set of material inputs (e.g., water, latrines, soap, food, fuel) and a set of culturally and socially appropriate messages needed to optimize the use of these materials. A primary tool for evaluating the efficacy of the services provided is environmental monitoring.

*Specific details on well and latrine construction can be found in other texts. *Public Health Engineering in Emergency Situation* (1994) by Medecins Sans Frontieres and *Environmental Health Engineering in the Tropics*, 2nd ed. by Cairncross S. and Feachem R. (John Wiley & Sons Ltd., 1993) are both excellent general texts for suggesting facility designs and guiding construction activities. Further information on vector control can be found in UNHCR's Vector Control in Refugee Situations PTSS/HCR, June 1996.

Bioterrorism

Bioterrorism is an emerging threat to the U.S. population. The bombings of the World Trade Center in New York City and the Murrah Federal Building in Oklahoma demonstrated to the public that terrorist activity within United States borders was a reality.[132] The likelihood of a chemical or biological warfare attack (CBW) is increasing according to a number of experts.[133] Defense Secretary William Cohen stated, "The threat is neither far fetched or far off...one that's only going to grow with time" and "The front lines are no longer overseas. It can just as well be in any American City."[133]

CBW agents can have an overwhelming impact on public health. On March 20, 1995, members of the Aum Shinriko religious cult released sarin, a nerve gas, in the Tokyo subway. Twelve people were killed, 1,000 required hospitalization, and 5,000 received medical attention.[133,134] In response to growing concerns for public safety, the Nunn-Lugar-Domenici Domestic Preparedness Program was established as part of the Defense Against Weapons of Mass Destruction Act of 1996.[135] This program was created to bolster emergency response levels at federal, state, and local levels but did not specifically address the role of public health.[132]

Although a new and demanding challenge for public health agencies, bioterrorism activity has significant historic antecedents and contemporary examples. In 1346, Tartar invaders attacked Kaffa (now Feodosia, Ukraine), a city defended by Genoese merchants. The Tartar invaders used bodies of plague victims to transmit disease by catapulting them over city walls. The plan was to spread the plague; indeed, the Genoese merchants contracted this disease, although it is unlikely the catapulting technique explained the transmission.[136,137] In 1763, Sir Jeffrey Amherst, commander of British troops in America, advocated the use of smallpox, writing: "Could it not be contrived to send the Small Pox among those Disaffected Tribes of Indians? We must on this occasion, use every Stratagem in our power to reduce them."[138]

More recently, in 1984, 715 individuals became ill after two members of an Oregon sect contaminated a salad bar at a local restaurant with *Salmonella typhimurium*, ostensibly to affect the outcome of a local election.[139] A wave of anthrax scares, all hoaxes so far, is now occurring and is stressing the capacity of local public health agencies to respond appropriately. Between April 1997 and June 1999, there were approximately 200 mailed or phoned bioterrorism threats, usually claiming that the contents could transmit anthrax.[140] As a result of these incidents, local emergency responders treated more than 13,000 potential victims, sometimes requiring these individuals to strip and undergo decontamination with bleach solutions.[140]

The CDC issued a report reviewing seven bioterrorism threats that occurred in 1998.[141] Again, most of these involved claims of anthrax, where laboratory tests showed no evidence of contamination by this agent.

A report by Garrett detailed one of these incidents in Wichita, Kansas. On August 18, 1998, several hundred workers were evacuated and a four-block area of downtown Wichita was cordoned off after a suspicious white powder was found in several stairwells and an elevator of an office building.[142] A threatening letter had been received in a manila envelope claiming that the substance was anthrax. Local emergency medical services and hazardous material units (HAZMAT) detained 200 potentially exposed individuals.

Testing for *B. anthracis* was performed by the U.S. Army Medical Research Institute of Infectious Diseases and a fluorescent antibody test and culture were negative. This situation reported in Wichita is far from an isolated incident, with similar scenarios in a growing number of communities.

Bioterrorism Agents

Some understanding of the specific agents that might be employed by terrorists will assist in adequate preparation for a bioterrorist incident.[136] The military weapons displayed in Table 4 and Exhibit 6 are helpful as a starting point. Of these, anthrax is most formidable in its production of mortality and is the agent of greatest concern (Table 5). Smallpox and pneumonic plague can also pose problems of magnitude and are contagious. Because the motives and thought processes of terrorists are difficult to understand, considering those agents that, if used, would produce the most serious consequences is advisable.[136] The CDC has developed such a list of critical agents for health preparedness (Table 6).[143] Category A has high impact and requires high preparedness. Category B has a lesser requirement for preparedness. Category C can be handled within current public health capacity.

Predictions of the agent used by bioterrorists are not possible, but taking the time to consider the spectrum of agents most likely to be used is helpful to public health practitioners in planning for preparedness and in developing protocols. Many of the diseases that may occur as a result of biologic terrorism are rare (inhalational anthrax, pneumonic plague) or have previously been globally eradicated (smallpox).[132] The possibly unannounced dissemination of a biologic agent may at first go unnoticed, with the exposed individuals leaving the scene and not showing signs of illness for hours, days, or weeks. This underscores the vital importance in investing in surveillance systems designed to capture local information. The first response to bioterrorism is at the local level, but subsequent public health management is coordinated at local, state, and federal levels.

The Threat List

The definition of the threat list depends heavily on who is being threatened and how the threat is perceived. The military definition focuses primarily on bacteriologic agents and toxins that have been weaponized in aerosol form by a nation to produce a large number of battlefield casualties. These are the prototypical weapons of mass destruction. The military's threat list is dynamic and depends on intelligence assessment. Thus, it is possible that an organism could be appropriate in theoretical terms as a threat but is not considered a threat because no one has developed a large-scale weapon for containment and dispersion.

The civilian threat list is much broader because the rapid onset or the effects of the diseases are not critical, and contagious diseases would also be considered effective bioterroristic agents. Many normal public health threats overlap with the agents of bioterrorism, both in the nature of the outbreaks produced, and in the nature of the response to control them. Pneumonic plague is a good example where a naturally occurring case generates a rapid and vigorous public health response to prevent further dissemination.

Table 4

Destroyed U.S. biological arsenal

Lethal Agents	Incapacitating Agents	Anti-crop Weapons
Bacillus anthracis	Venezuelan equine encephalitis	Wheat-stem rust
Botulinum toxin	Staphylococcal enterotoxin B	Rye-stem rust
Francisella tularensis	*Brucella suis*	Rice-blast spore
	Coxiella burnetii	

Source: Reprinted from *U.S. Army Activity in the U.S. Biological Warfare Programs,* Pub. No. B193427L, 1997, Washington, DC: U.S. Department of the Army.

For purposes of this discussion, it is clear that there are relative priorities among the diseases being classified and that there are only three major categories of agents. Within these three categories, only five agents (anthrax, smallpox, plague, botulism, and tularemia) are considered serious threats. The first category of disease is that caused by an aerosolized release of bacteria. This produces respiratory or pulmonary disease. The three agents in this category are anthrax, plague, and tularemia. A second category of illness is where the dissemination is dependent on person-to-person transmission, such as smallpox. The third category of disease is that caused by contamination of food, water, or other ingested material, such as botulinum toxin.

Exhibit 6

Rating system (Russian) of bioagent distribution according to probability of use as BW

- Smallpox virus
- *Yersinia pestis*
- *Bacillus anthracis*
- Botulinum toxin
- Venezuelan equine encephalitis virus
- *Francisella tularensis*
- *Coxiella burnetii*
- Marburg virus
- Influenza virus
- *Burkholderia mallei*
- *Rickettsia typhi*

Source: Reprinted from A.A. Vorobjev et al., Key Problems of Controlling Especially Dangerous Infections, in *Proceedings of an International Symposium: Severe Infectious Diseases: Epidemiology, Express-Diagnostics and Prevention,* 1997, State Scientific Institution, Volgo-Vyatsky Center of Applied Biotechnology, Kirov, Russia.

Anthrax is considered, both in the scientific and popular literature, to be a highly efficacious biologic warfare agent for a number of reasons. First, it forms spores, which give it stability in aerosol. Second, it is relatively easy to disseminate using off-the-shelf technology. Third, if acquired by the respiratory route, the disease is frequently fatal. There are difficulties in preparing a form of the agent that is stable in aerosol, but these difficulties were apparently overcome in the course of the former Soviet Union's program, and it is possible that well-informed terrorists could replicate those procedures.

Smallpox, as mentioned previously, has the additional feature of being highly contagious in unimmunized populations, with a cycle of 10 to 14 days, an attack rate of up to 90 percent, and mortality as high as 35 percent. What makes this disease a less likely threat is that an eradication program eliminated the natural illness from the planet and only two samples of live virus remain: One is under the control of the United States at the CDC and the other is held by Russia. Some experts, therefore, consider that it would be hard for a terrorist to acquire live smallpox virus. However, it was reported in the *New York Times* (1999) that smallpox virus is held by Iraq and North Korea in addition to the two approved sites. Uncertainty underscores the potential threat and the fact that international agreements cannot be relied upon.

Plague, a respiratory-acquired illness, is also spread person-to-person. Because it occurs as an en-

Table 5

Results of the hypothetical aerosol dissemination of various infecting agents

Agent	Downwind Carriage	Deaths	Total Casualties
Venezuelan Equine Encephalitis	1 km	400	35,000
Tick-Borne Encephalitis	1 km	9,500	35,000
Epidemic Typhus	5 km	19,000	85,000
Brucellosis	10 km	500	100,000
Plague	10 km	55,000	100,000
Q-Fever	>20 km	150	125,000
Tularemia	>20 km	30,000	125,000
Anthrax	>>20 km	95,000	125,000

Note: Casualty figures assume 50 kg of dried agent disseminated along a 2-km line upwind of a population center of 500,000.
Source: Data from *Health Aspects of Chemical and Biological Weapons*, © 1970, World Health Organization.

zootic disease of rodents in the United States, it may be possible to obtain an isolate for use as a terrorist agent. Botulism is likewise an environmental organism that can be easily cultured from soil. Its toxin has the disturbing clinical feature of necessitating intensive supportive care of its victims. Additionally, the treatment for it, in the form of an antitoxin, is limited in supply and availability.

Tularemia can be disseminated in water. In aerosol form it produces a severely debilitating pneumonia but without as high mortality as anthrax. Other agents are on longer threat lists. Q fever and brucella produce, in most instances, mild illnesses that would not generate large-scale stress on medical systems or produce large-scale panic. The agents in the next rank of concern are regular public health threats such as viral encephalitis, cholera, salmonella, influenza, and staphylococcal enterotoxin B.

Differences between Overt and Covert Release

It is unlikely that terrorists would use an overt release, in the form of an announced event or some-

Table 6

Critical agents for health preparedness

Category A	Category B	Category C
Variola virus	*Coxiella burnetii*	All other biological agents may emerge as future threats to public health
Bacillus anthracis	*Brucellae*	
Yersinia pestis	*Burkholderia mallei*	
Botulinum toxin	*Burkholderia pseudomallei*	
Francisella tularensis	Alphaviruses	
Filoviruses and arenaviruses	*Rickettsia prowezekii*	
	Certain toxins (Ricin, SEB)	
	Chlamydia psittaci	
	Food safety threat agents (*Salmonellae*, *E coli* O157:H7)	
	Water safety threat agents (*Vibrio cholera*, etc)	

Source: Reprinted from *Critical Agents for Health Preparedness, Summary of Selection Process and Recommendations*, Centers for Disease Control and Prevention, National Center for Infectious Diseases, 1999.

thing that is recognized at the time, as their mode for biologic terrorism. This type of release would allow treatment before the onset of disease. There are now examples where the management of biologic threats has changed significantly. In the case of overt releases, an assessment of the threat is made before the response is initiated. In many cases, announced biologic threats are considered hoaxes, and a limited and tempered response is activated. A limited response in these cases does not represent a casual response on the part of law enforcement, but rather a sophisticated analysis of the situation that allows a resolution of the incident without major difficulties.

A covert release of a biologic agent will present as illness in the community, and its detection is dependent on traditional surveillance methods. Recent federal programs have emphasized enhancing such systems and increasing the sensitivity of frontline medical practitioners to the importance of recognizing and reporting suspicious syndromes. The covert release of a contagious agent has the potential for large-scale spread before detection. A release in an airport or in a highly mobile population could disseminate a pathogen such as smallpox throughout most of the world before the epidemic would be recognized. To bring this potential epidemic under control, a major multifocal international response would need to be activated. In the case of anthrax, the treatment can be time-sensitive. If individuals are already exhibiting severe symptoms, treatment is often not effective.

Local Health Department Response

LHDs are first-line responders for incidents of bioterrorism, requiring planning for preparedness. Preparedness at the local level includes readiness assessment, expansion of surveillance and epidemiology capacity, and provisions for laboratory identification of the chemical/biologic agent.[142] Development of protocols is recommended to deal with the most likely agents to be encountered. In addition, training of personnel is needed. The foremost consideration is effective and preplanned strategies for communication with other community agencies and the public.

In planning a response strategy, LHDs should identify key responders in the community, including emergency medical services, HAZMAT, and police and fire agencies. Discussions should also take place with the directors of emergency services at local hospitals and the poison control center. In these incidents, individuals may appear at their local hospital with concerns about potential exposure. Uniform protocols between institutions, particularly with respect to prophylactic antibiotic usage, are advisable.

Linkages with a laboratory with the capability to identify agents of concern, the state public health agency, and the CDC should be accomplished in advance of any reported incident. A surveillance system to track the large numbers of potentially exposed individuals is needed and can be designed in accord with the guidance described earlier in this chapter. Methods for secure communication need to be explored. Advance discussions with the media are also advisable because extensive television, radio, and newspaper coverage of these incidents can provoke copycat episodes. In a number of recent instances, dissemination of the news has been delayed by the media in an effort to forestall repeat incidents.

The Federal Response

The Nunn-Lugar Funds provide training and equipment to 120 major cities in the United States.

Congress also provided for the establishment of Metropolitan Medical Response Systems under the public health system. These are assets that would be activated in a disaster situation involving either chemical or biologic weapons. The early federal response is deemed appropriate for a chemical event recognized by people becoming acutely ill. If terrorists wanted to have impact using biologic weapons, the last thing they would want is for the attack to be recognized and appropriate countermeasures applied, which would severely blunt the attack.

The most serious difficulty with the early federal response is that state and local public health authorities were not involved in establishment of the response systems, and the discussions were held almost exclusively in the emergency response environment. This is a problem because a biologic event would most likely present as the occurrence of a cluster of an unusual disease in the population, and the entities traditionally responsible for recognizing and responding to such an event are public health organizations. The response required for a biologic event is totally dissimilar to that required for an overt chemical event where fire, police, or HAZMAT units are the key part of the response. If a release of a contagious disease such as smallpox occurred, a number of patients would appear in emergency departments with rash illnesses that would be reported to authorities as suspect smallpox. A public health response, including quarantine and immunization, could then be activated.

National Program for the Public Health Response to Bioterrorism

Prior to fiscal year 1999/2000, no specific federal funds were set aside for a public health response to bioterrorism. In fiscal year 1999/2000, a $179 million program was established under the sponsorship of Senator Lauch Faircloth from North Carolina. The program included a significant component for central DHHS activities, and the remaining $121 million was specifically earmarked for the CDC. Approximately $51 million is allocated to a National Pharmaceutical Stockpile to detect, diagnose, and treat illnesses caused by potential bioterrorism pathogens.[132] This initiative will assist in coordinating a response and communication between local, state, and federal levels of public health and other response agencies.

A new activity was established at the CDC called the Biological Preparedness and Response Program (BPRP). During the planning, a partnership of BPRP and state and local public health programs formulated into a five-part program for the remaining $70 million. The five components of the program are planning, surveillance and epidemiologic response, a biologic laboratory network, a chemical laboratory response capability, and a health alert network. The CDC is developing public health guidelines to assist local public health agencies in developing bioterrorism preparedness plans and response protocols. These include self-assessment tools for preparedness, proficiency testing programs, attack simulation programs, and computerized resource-tracking systems. The CDC awarded $1.5 million to nine states and two cities in 1999 for preparedness and response enhancement with plans for additional funding to other jurisdictions in the following 3–5 years.[132]

The national disease surveillance systems are being upgraded to include biologic and chemical agents. In 1999, to improve state and local surveillance activities, the CDC awarded $7.8 million to 31 states and 3 large cities with further funding planned. The CDC and its public health partners are also establishing a Laboratory Response Network for Bioterrorism that will link 50 states and additional localities. The CDC has awarded a total of approximately $8.8 million in grants to 41 states and 2 large city health laboratories to improve capacity for identifying biologic agents. The CDC has also created an internal Rapid Response and Advanced Technology Laboratory to provide 24-hour availability for diagnoses of illnesses potentially secondary to agents of biologic terrorism.[132]

In developing this program, the CDC called together a group of external advisors who reviewed the biologic threat list from the public health standpoint. This advisory group reaffirmed the five highest priority agents previously mentioned and added viral hemorrhagic fevers. It also designated a second tier of organisms, for which protocols for testing are in the final stages of development.

The CDC program resulted in awards to 41 jurisdictions in the late fall of 1999. The planning component has a limited number of awards and is designed to develop templates for biologic response programs in small, medium, and large jurisdictions. The surveillance and response program, which is considered by many to be the key to the overall success of the project, includes such things as active surveillance for threat diseases, adding threat diseases to the list of reportable diseases, instituting electronic laboratory reporting, and adding staff to respond rapidly in the event of a suspected outbreak of one of these unusual diseases. The biologic laboratory network will be described in specific detail later in this chapter. The chemical laboratory network is intended to provide backup to the CDC in the event of overload. This is based on the assumption that a chemical incident would result in an expanded need for both diagnostic tests to aid in exposure assessments and medical follow-up of exposed individuals. To date, the CDC has funded four laboratories and provided mass spectrometry instruments to them.

The CDC is also building a Health Alert Network (HAN) to communicate with state and local health agencies. The HAN is the connection of all public health officers to the Internet. Under this program, a secure Web site will be established, and individuals will be trained to facilitate their effective use of this system. This national communications and distance-learning network will include high-capacity, continuous Internet connections for secure electronic communications and Web access with the ability to participate in distance learning and to receive information and guidance on bioterrorism threats. This project has the largest budget of the five program components. The CDC distributed $19 million in 1999 to state and local health departments for the development of the HAN.[132]

The Public Health Laboratory Network

The laboratory response network for bioterrorism is a CDC-sponsored program with network coordination by contract with the Association of Public Health Laboratories. All levels of laboratories are connected with built-in redundancy. The system emphasizes rapid turnaround and accuracy. The laboratories are the central points of contact for technology validation and transfer. A scientific steering group, in collaboration with the CDC, will be developing and defining priorities and protocols for new technology.

The network of public health laboratories is extensive, consisting of a program in each state and in many local jurisdictions. Using California as the example, the network concept is based on the idea of specialization rather than regionalization. There are 39 free-standing county laboratories, each with a broad range in capability and support. The local laboratories' infrastructure has undergone decay in the last few years, but they are well organized for certain things. Examples that are working in the state include the testing by one laboratory for tickborne diseases in an area of endemic occurrence, the delegation of HIV viral burden to seven major counties with the highest volume, and the establishment of computer support for rapid logistics and communication that would be an essential element of a network for response to bioterrorism as well.

The most important reason for establishing a network of public health laboratories to assist in the response to bioterrorism is that all the diseases that are threats occur naturally in the United States. For example, botulism, plague, anthrax, tularemia, and poxvirus illnesses are routinely evaluated by many public health laboratories. Not only do these diseases occur with some frequency, but the public health laboratories are in almost all cases primarily responsible for their diagnosis. While the frequency of these diseases is low, the impact is high because of the speed with which these diseases spread (i.e., pneumatic plague). The frequency of current testing is not low, and in California alone, requests for botulism testing of humans occur twice a week.

The other major premise behind establishing the network is that standard or classical microbiology technique works well for the major threat agents. The current methods of detecting bacterial agents (gram stain, culture on selective media, visual colony morphology, growth after heat shock, and confirmatory methods using phage and direct immunofluorescence) are well established for definitive recognition and diagnosis. In the case of virology, methods such as isolation in cell culture, inoculation of animals, direct fluorescence methods, and electron microscopy are well established as definitive methods.

The public health laboratory network for response to bioterrorism has four levels of performance defined as A, B, C, and D. Level A performance, in the case of bacteriology, is culture only in clinical and small public health laboratories. Level B performance is first-level confirmation using direct fluorescence or phage testing, for example. Major county and small state public health laboratories fill this role. Level C laboratories provide the second level of confirmation with more complicated methods including molecular diagnostics and are major state public health laboratories. A key task of level C laboratories in the future will be to validate new technology and pass it down to level B laboratories. Level D laboratories are federal and private partners in the Public Health Service, Department of Defense, national laboratories, and industry that can perform research on and development of new techniques for passing down to the lower levels of the network.

The laboratory network has five major tasks. The network was established to enhance the capability of level A laboratories by providing training to bench-level microbiologists in the use of algorithms so that suspect key organisms are not ignored or discarded. The network will deploy confirmatory reagents from a central stockpile to level B labs using predominantly fluorescence and phage methodology at present. Reagents will be prepared and in some cases distributed by level C laboratories, and new technology will be validated in level C laboratories, and transferred to level B laboratories after field testing. Research will be conducted in level D laboratories. Finally, a contract with the Association of Public

Health Laboratories has been established to coordinate logistics and communication. This includes a secure Web site for registering laboratories, obtaining protocols, and ordering reagents. In the future, reporting of suspect threat diseases also may be done over the Internet.

This can foster the level D laboratories doing the research and development that is so important as an underpinning for this field. The laboratory network can partner with Department of Justice programs to handle environmental samples. Early in the development of this program, protocols were rapidly developed, sent around for comment, and made available on the secure Web site. The next step will be the provision of hands-on training, in some cases at the state level, and in other cases at the CDC.

If a covert event that is not recognized immediately occurs, how is the connection with the laboratory made? The occurrence of disease in the community would trigger the public health control programs to submit samples to the laboratory and report to the surveillance network. In the event of an announced threat or an overt event, the event would be reported to the Federal Bureau of Investigation (FBI), and the FBI would bring samples to the nearest appropriate laboratory resource in the network. In the case of such events, the FBI will make the determination of which laboratory will be involved.

There are four advantages for using the procedures of a public health laboratory program. First, existing tests give definitive results. Second, the procedures that are used are validated under the license of the laboratory and can be readily adapted to environmental samples such as might happen after an overt threat, or in the attribution of a source of a sample. Third, the laboratories are all certified under the Clinical Laboratory Improvement Act or CLIA, with appropriate quality assurance and quality control procedures. Finally, the personnel are highly skilled and familiar with following complex algorithms.

Using existing public health laboratories to respond to bioterrorism also has limitations. First, the final result is usually not available for a day or two, but preliminary results can be available in minutes or hours. In particular, the minimum response time for a definitive negative result with a rapidly growing organism such as anthrax may be 16 hours. More slowly growing organisms or complex procedures may take 48 hours or more. Second, these methods require a fixed laboratory facility and these techniques are not readily adaptable to a field situation.

What Is the Status of Rapid Tests?

One question that comes up frequently is what is the status of the commercial rapid hand-held assays for detection of biologic agents because the early federal response involved their purchase and dissemination. These assays are based on antibody capture technology from the 1970s and suffer from the fact that their sensitivity is not as good as culture or molecular methods by three logs or more. The specificity of these methods with stimulants has not been determined, and they can be confounded by commonly used pesticides or killed organisms. Therefore, such tests cannot be used in decision making because the sensitivity does not allow one to exclude the possibility of an event and nonspecificity does not allow one to call an event definitely. The network will evaluate and attempt to qualify these rapid test methods and for future use where appropriate.

What Countermeasures Are Available?

Preventive measures performed before the occurrence of the bioterrorist event have distinct advantages. Unfortunately, large-scale immunization of the population for smallpox has been discontinued. The response to the reintroduction of smallpox, natural or unnatural, would be a rapid large-scale immunization program to surround the outbreak. This is similar to what was done in the eradication campaign of the late 1970s. One difficulty with this strategy is that there is a limited supply of vaccine, approximately 50 million doses worldwide, and the vaccine is aging. There are plans to make a new product. This initiative has been stalled for the past few years but appears to be moving forward again. There are serious questions about how it could be licensed because there are no natural infections to prevent to conduct an efficacy trial. There are difficulties in its administration. Vaccinators require specialized training in the use of bifurcated needles. Prescreening of vaccinees for HIV may be required to prevent the occurrence of disseminated vaccinia in such immunocompromised individuals. The smallpox vaccine also has a small but significant number of complications that require the availability of an immune globulin. Vaccinia immune globulin is also in short supply and there are difficulties with plans for making more in the future.

For the major bacterial threat agents, the administration of antibiotics is the key component of the response. In the event of a release of anthrax, there are a number of possible scenarios for the large-scale administration of antibiotics. Dosing could start with the antibiotic ciprofloxacin to be replaced by penicillin once antibiotic susceptibility is determined. (The definition of the public health response to anthrax and full discussion of the use of antibiotics including use in pregnancy and pediatrics, is found in a white paper published by a working group of the Johns Hopkins Center for Civilian Biodefense in the *Journal of the American Medical Association.*) A licensed vaccine for anthrax has been administrated fairly widely to military populations. Administration of this vaccine to at-risk individuals after release of anthrax would cut down on the time of antibiotic administration required.

Antibiotics are the mainstay of the response to plague and tularemia. The description of the response to these organisms, including detail antibiotic usage, is found in the Johns Hopkins Center white papers on these particular organisms. The public health response to a botulism outbreak is a bit more complicated because the occurrence of paralysis in a number of individuals may overrun the short supply of both ventilators and intensive care beds in pulmonary units. Further, the immune globulin used in the routine treatment of both wound and foodborne botulism is in short supply, and increasing the supply would require a major effort to manufacture a large enough stockpile.

Part of the federal public health response to this problem has been the earmarking of a significant amount of money for a national stock of antibiotics and vaccine for the major bioterrorist agents of threat. The first phase of this program came online at the beginning of the year 2000. The long-term strategy for this program includes developing a "virtual supply" by contracting with manufacturers to provide large amounts of product on relatively short notice. Although this supply is called a stockpile, massive amounts of antibiotics will not actually be centrally stored.

Recent well-documented shortages of penicillin in the United States have alerted planners about the availability of antibiotics. In addition, the precursors of some antibiotics are not produced in the United States and may require the cooperation of foreign governments in the event large amounts of drugs are needed on short notice.

Appropriateness of Public Health Program for Bioterrorism Response

Cohen and colleagues[144] suggested that biologic warfare is "public health in reverse," because biologic warfare causes disease, and public health is the profession dedicated to preventing and treating disease. They suggested that the federal preparedness programs, described earlier in the chapter, are equivalent to biologic warfare itself because of the emphasis on the military response and the diversion "of resources from other, more urgently needed public health tasks." These authors claim that funding for bioterrorist initiatives has increased at the expense of existing public health budgets. However, considering the potential threat, and the fact that bioterrorism could occur anywhere, preparedness is the prudent action. Criticism of preparedness fails to acknowledge and factor in the new money that has gone to the CDC to support preparedness and response to biologic terrorism. The funds that are in this program are earmarked for dual use and will support general preparedness, response to epidemics, surveillance of syndromes, and rapid epidemiologic evaluation. In total, this program will benefit the recognition and control of many diseases of public health importance, in addition to supporting preparedness for diseases due to bioterroristic activities. It is difficult to see how this program could be anything other than a win for public health.

■ ■ ■

Public health organizations carry out a broad and complex set of responsibilities in preparing for and responding to disasters and acts of bioterrorism. Carrying out these responsibilities requires a multi-organizational effort. Disaster epidemiology and assessment are important components of the public health response, as these activities support scientific investigation as well as disaster management decision making. Public health organizations also play critical roles in preventing and controlling the psychosocial effects of disasters. The emerging threat of bioterrorism calls attention to the importance of public health organizations in disaster preparedness and response initiatives, creating new risks and responsibilities for organizations along the continuum of public health practice settings. The contemporary public health environment demands informed decision making and effective management in response to the health threats posed by manmade and natural disasters.

REFERENCES

1. S.W.A. Gunn, *Multilingual Dictionary of Disaster Medicine and International Relief* (Dordrecht, The Netherlands: Kluwer Academic Publishers, 1990).
2. P. Showalter and M.F. Myers, "Natural Disasters in the United States as Release Agents of Oil, Chemicals, or Radiological Materials between 1980–1989," *Risk Analysis* 14 (1994): 169–182.
3. F. Cuny, "Introduction to Disaster Management: Lesson 2—Concepts and Terms in Disaster Management," *Prehospital Disaster Medicine* 8 (1993): 89–94.
4. *Robert T. Stafford Disaster Relief and Emergency Assistance Act,* Public Law 93–288.
5. E. Auf der Heide, *Community Medical Disaster Planning and Evaluation Guide* (Dallas, TX: American College of Emergency Physicians, 1996).
6. E.L. Quarantelli, *Delivery of Emergency Medical Care in Disasters: Assumptions and Realities* (New York: Irvington Publishers, Inc., 1983).
7. S.P. Nishenko and G.A. Bollinger, "Forecasting Damaging Earthquakes in the Central and Eastern United States," *Science* 249 (1990): 1,412–1,416.
8. W.M. Gray, "Strong Association between West African Rainfall and US Landfall of Intense Hurricanes," *Science* 249 (1990): 1,251–1,256.
9. Universite Catholique de Louvain, Brussels, Belguim, "EM-DAT: The Office of Foreign Disaster Assistance/CRED International Disaster Database." http://www.md.ucl.ac.be/cred. Accessed 20 April 2000.
10. National Research Council, *Reducing Disasters' Toll: The US Decade for Natural Disaster Reduction* (Washington, DC: National Academy Press, 1989).
11. L.R. Johnston Associates, *Floodplain Management in the United States: An Assessment Report. Volume 2 Full Report. Prepared for the Federal Interagency Floodplain Management Taskforce. FIA-18/June 1992* (Washington, DC: U.S. Federal Emergency Management Agency, Federal Interagency Floodplain Management Taskforce, 1992).
12. P.R. Berke and T. Beatley, *Planning for Earthquakes* (Baltimore: The Johns Hopkins Press, 1992).
13. J.E. Beavers, Testimony of Dr. James E. Beavers, Member, Scientific Advisory Committee of the National Center for Earthquake Engineering Research, State University of New York at Buffalo, Buffalo, NY. Testimony before the Committee on Science, Space, and Technology. U.S. House of Representatives. One Hundred First Congress First Session November 17, 1989 (No. 101). Washington, DC: U.S. Government Printing Office, 92–95.
14. Utah Earthquake Preparedness Information Center, *Earthquakes: What You Should Know When Living in Utah* (Salt Lake City, UT: Federal Emergency Management Agency).
15. T.J. Culliton et al., *50 Years of Population Change along the Nation's Coasts, 1960–2010* (Coastal Trends Series, Report 2) (Rockville, MD: National Oceanic and Atmospheric Administration, 1990).
16. C. Axelrod et al., "Primary Health Care and the Midwest Flood Disaster," *Public Health Reports 109,* no. 5 (1994): 601–605.
17. K. Gautam, "Organizational Problems Faced by the Missouri DOH in Providing Disaster Relief during the 1993 Floods," *Journal of Public Health Management and Practice 4,* no. 4 (1998): 79–86.
18. C.A. Evans, "Public Health Impact of the 1992 Los Angeles Unrest," *Public Health Reports 108,* no. 3 (1993): 265–272.
19. "Health Topics A to Z." http://www.cdc.gov/health/diseases.htm. (31 May 2000) Accessed 15 June 2000.
20. S. Whitman et al., "Mortality in Chicago Attributed to the July 1995 Heat Wave," *American Journal of Public Health 87,* no. 9 (1997): 1,515–1,518.
21. R. Lyskowski and S. Rice, *The Big One: Hurricane Andrew* (Kansas City, MO: The Miami Herald Publishing Co., 1992).
22. S.J. Carr et al., "The Public Health Response to the Los Angeles 1994 Earthquake," *American Journal of Public Health 86,* no. 4 (1996): 589–590.
23. E. Noji, ed., *The Public Health Consequences of Disaster* (New York: Oxford University Press, 1997).
24. L.F. Saylor and J.E. Gordon, "The Medical Component of Natural Disasters," *American Journal of the Medical Sciences* 234 (1957): 342–362.
25. A.S. Buist and R.S. Bernstein, eds., "Health Effects of Volcanoes: An Approach to Evaluating the Health Effects of an Environmental Hazard," *American Journal of Public Health 76,* no. 3 (suppl.) (1986): 1–90.
26. R.S. Bernstein et al., "Immediate Public Health Concerns and Actions in Volcanic Eruptions: Lessons from Mount St. Helens Eruptions, May 18–October 18, 1980," *American Journal of Public Health 76,* no. 3 (suppl.) (1986): 25–37.
27. Resolution 44/236 of the General Assembly of the United Nations, 1989.
28. Resolution 54/219 of the General Assembly of the United Nations.
29. L.Y. Landesman, ed., *Emergency Preparedness in the Healthcare Environment* (Oakbrook, IL: Joint Commission on Accreditation of Healthcare Organizations, 1997).
30. H.M. Ginzburg et al., "The Public Health Services Response to Hurricane Andrew," *Public Health Reports 108,* no. 2 (1993): 241–244.
31. P. Lewis, *Final Report: Governor's Disaster Planning and Response Review Committee* (Tallahassee, FL: Governor's Disaster Planning and Response Review Committee, 1993).

32. L.Y. Landesman, "The Availability of Disaster Preparation Courses at US Schools of Public Health," *American Journal of Public Health 83,* no. 10 (1993): 1,494–1,495.
33. Office of Disease Prevention and Health Promotion, U.S. Department of Health and Human Services, *Healthy People 2010* (Washington, DC: 1998). http://www.health.gov/healthypeople.
34. P.W. O'Carroll et al., "The Rapid Implementation of a Statewide Emergency Health Information System during the 1993 Iowa Flood," *American Journal of Public Health 85,* no. 4 (1995): 564–567.
35. Joint Commission on Accreditation of Healthcare Organizations, *Comprehensive Accreditation Manual for Hospitals: The Official Handbook* (EC 1.6, EC 2.5, EC 2.9, EC-5, EC-6, EC-12, EC-13, EC-25, EC-26, EC-49, EC-50) (Oakbrook Terrace, IL: 2000).
36. R. Bissell et al., "Health Care Personnel in Disaster Response: Reversible Roles or Territorial Imperatives?" *Emergency Medicine Clinics of North America 14,* no. 2 (1996): 267–288.
37. A. Kuehl, ed., *Prehospital Systems and Medical Oversight* (St. Louis, MO: Mosby, 1994).
38. T.E. Drabek et al., *Managing Multiorganizational Emergency Response: Emergency Research and Rescue Networks in Natural Disaster and Remote Area Setting* (Boulder, CO: Natural Hazards Information Center, University of Colorado, 1981).
39. E. Auf der Heide, *Disaster Response: Principles of Preparation and Coordination* (St. Louis, MO: C.V. Mosby, 1981).
40. "United States Government: Federal Response Plan (For Public Law 93–288, as Amended), April, 1992." [Publication no. 9230.1-PL] (Washington, DC: U.S. Government Printing Office, 1999).
41. F. Cuny, "Introduction to Disaster Management, Lesson 1: The Scope of Disaster Management," *Prehospital and Disaster Medicine 7,* no. 4 (1992): 400–409.
42. A. Ahlbom and S. Norell, *Introduction to Modern Epidemiology* (Chestnut Hill, MA: Epidemiology Resources, Inc., 1984).
43. M.F. Lechat, "The Epidemiology of Disasters," *Proceedings of the Royal Society of Medicine* 69 (1976): 421–426.
44. Reserved.
45. C. Bern et al., "Risk Factors for Mortality in the Bangladesh Cyclone of 1991," *Bulletin of the World Health Organization* 71 (1993): 73–78.
46. P.J. Baxter et al., "Mount St. Helens Eruptions: The Acute Respiratory Effects of Volcanic Ash in a North American Community," *Archives of Environmental Health* 38 (1983): 138–143.
47. U.S. Centers for Disease Control and Prevention, "Needs Assessment Following Hurricane Georges–Dominican Republic, 1998," *Morbidity and Mortality Weekly Report* 48 (1999): 93–95.
48. M. Anker, "Epidemiological and Statistical Methods for Rapid Health Assessment: Introduction," *World Health Statistics Quarterly* 44 (1991): 94–97.
49. S.B. Thacker and R.L. Berkelman, "Public Health Surveillance in the United States," *Epidemiology Review* 10 (1988): 164–190.
50. S.F. Wetterhall and E.K. Noji, "Surveillance and Epidemiology," in *The Public Health Consequences of Disasters,* ed. E.K. Noji (New York: Oxford University Press, 1997), 37–64.
51. Pan American Health Organization, *Humanitarian Supply Management System* (Washington, DC: 1998). http://www.disaster.info.desastres.net/SUMA. Accessed 18 April 2000.
52. U.S. Agency for International Development, *Famine Early Warning* System (Washington, DC: 1985). http://www.info.usaid.gov/fews/fews.html. Accessed 18 April 2000.
53. R.I. Glass and E.K. Noji, "Epidemiologic Surveillance Following Disasters," in *Public Health Surveillance,* eds. W. Halperin and E.L. Baker (New York: Van Nostrand Reinhold, 1992), 195–205.
54. U.S. Centers for Disease Control and Prevention, Epidemiology Program Office, "Training Notes" (Atlanta, GA: 1992).
55. P.J. Baxter et al., "Mount St. Helens Eruptions, May 18 to June 12, 1980: An Overview of the Acute Health Impact," *Journal of the American Medical Association* 246 (1988): 2,585–2,589.
56. P. Duclos, *American Red Cross Disaster Database Collaborative Project: Surveillance System for Natural Disasters Using American Red Cross Records* (Atlanta, GA: U.S. Centers for Disease Control and Prevention, 1988).
57. J.H. van Bemmel and M.A. Musen, eds., *Handbook of Medical Informatics* (Houten, the Netherlands: Bohn Stafleu Van Loghum, 1997).
58. E.T. Gerrity and B.W. Flynn, "Mental Health Consequences of Disasters," in *Public Health Consequences of Disasters,* ed. E.K. Noji (New York: Oxford University Press, 1997), 101–121.
59. D. Myers, *Disaster Response and Recovery: A Handbook for Mental Health Professionals* (Rockville, MD: Center for Mental Health Services, 1994).
60. R.J. Ursano et al., "Trauma and Disaster," in *Individual and Community Responses to Trauma and Disaster: The Structure of Human Chaos,* eds. R.J. Ursano et al. (Cambridge, England: Cambridge University Press, 1994), 3–27.
61. K.J. Tierney, *Disaster Preparedness and Response: Research Findings and Guidance from the Social Science Literature* (Preliminary Paper #193) (Newark, DE: Disaster Research Center, University of Delaware, 1993).
62. B.H. Young et al., *Disaster Mental Health Services: A Guidebook for Clinicians and Administrators* (Menlo Park, CA: National Center for Post-Traumatic Stress Disorder, 1998).
63. E.T. Gerrity and P. Steinglass, "Relocation Stress Following Natural Disasters," in *Individual and Community Responses to Trauma and Disaster: The Structure of Human Chaos,* eds. R.J. Ursano et al. (Cambridge, England: Cambridge University Press, 1994), 220–247.
64. P.E. Hodgkinson and M. Stewart, *Coping with Catastrophe: A Handbook of Post-Disaster Psychosocial Aftercare,* 2d ed. (London: Routledge, 1998).

65. R. Janoff-Bulman, "The Aftermath of Victimization: Rebuilding Shattered Assumptions," in *Trauma and Its Wake: The Study and Treatment of Post-Traumatic Stress Disorder*, ed. C.R. Figley (New York: Brunner/Mazel Publishers, 1985), 15–35.
66. S.A. Murphy, "Health and Recovery Status of Victims One and Three Years Following a Natural Disaster," in *Trauma and Its Wake: Traumatic Stress Theory, Research, and Intervention*, ed. C.R. Figley (New York: Brunner/Mazel Publishers, 1986), 133–155.
67. *Training Manual for Human Service Workers in Major Disasters* (Washington, DC: Center for Mental Health Services, Substance Abuse and Mental Health Services Administration, U.S. Department of Health and Human Services, 1978, 1996).
68. D.M. Hartsough and D.G. Myers, *Disaster Work and Mental Health: Prevention and Control of Stress among Workers* (Washington, DC: Center for Mental Health Services, Substance Abuse and Mental Health Services Administration, U.S. Public Health Service, 1995).
69. C.R. Figley, "Traumatic Stress: The Role of the Family and Social Support System," in *Trauma and Its Wake: Traumatic Stress Theory, Research, and Intervention*, ed. C.R. Figley (New York: Brunner/Mazel Publishers, 1986), 39–54.
70. S.E. Hobfoll et al., "Conservation of Resources and Traumatic Stress," in *Traumatic Stress: From Theory to Practice*, eds. J.R. Freedy and S.E. Hobfoll (New York: Plenum Press, 1995), 29–47.
71. E.G. Karam, "Comorbidity of Posttraumatic Stress Disorder and Depression," in *Posttraumatic Stress Disorder: Acute and Long-Term Responses to Trauma and Disaster*, eds. C.S. Fullerton and R.J. Ursano (Washington, DC: American Psychiatric Press, 1997), 77–90.
72. K.J. Hoffman and J.E. Sasaki, "Comorbidity of Substance Abuse and PTSD," in *Posttraumatic Stress Disorder: Acute and Long-Term Responses to Trauma and Disaster*, eds. C.S. Fullerton and R.J. Ursano (Washington, DC: American Psychiatric Press, 1997), 159–174.
73. American Psychiatric Association, *Diagnostic and Statistical Manual of Mental Disorders*, 4th ed. (DSM-IV) (Washington, DC: 1994).
74. G. DeGirolamo and A.C. McFarlane, "The Epidemiology of PTSD: A Comprehensive Review of the International Literature," in *Ethnocultural Aspects of Posttraumatic Stress Disorder: Issues, Research, and Clinical Applications*, eds. A.J. Marsella et al. (Washington, DC: American Psychological Association, 1996), 33–85.
75. C.S. Fullerton and R.J. Ursano, eds., *Posttraumatic Stress Disorder: Acute and Long-Term Responses to Trauma and Disaster* (Washington, DC: American Psychiatric Press, 1997), 3–18.
76. L.S. O'Brien, *Traumatic Events and Mental Health* (Cambridge, England: Cambridge University Press, 1998).
77. C.S. Fullerton and R.J. Ursano, "Posttraumatic Responses in Spouse/Significant Others of Disaster Workers," in *Posttraumatic Stress Disorder: Acute and Long-Term Responses to Trauma and Disaster*, eds. C.S. Fullerton and R.J. Ursano (Washington, DC: American Psychiatric Press, 1997), 59–75.
78. A.J. Marsella et al., eds. *Ethnocultural Aspects of Posttraumatic Stress Disorder: Issues, Research, and Clinical Applications* (Washington, DC: American Psychological Association, 1996).
79. B.L. Green, "Cross-National and Ethnocultural Issues in Disaster Research," in *Ethnocultural Aspects of Posttraumatic Stress Disorder: Issues, Research, and Clinical Applications*, eds. A.J. Marsella et al. (Washington, DC: American Psychological Association, 1996), 341–361.
80. M.J. Friedman and A.J. Marsella, "Posttraumatic Stress Disorder: An Overview of the Concept," in *Ethnocultural Aspects of Posttraumatic Stress Disorder: Issues, Research, and Clinical Applications*, eds. A.J. Marsella et al. (Washington, DC: American Psychological Association, 1996), 11–32.
81. F.D. Gusman et al., "A Multicultural Approach and Developmental Framework for Treating Trauma," in *Ethnocultural Aspects of Posttraumatic Stress Disorder: Issues, Research, and Clinical Applications* (Washington, DC: American Psychological Association, 1996), 439–457.
82. K. Erikson, *Everything in Its Path: Destruction of Community in the Buffalo Creek Flood* (New York: Simon & Schuster, 1976).
83. B.L. Green et al., "Buffalo Creek Survivors in the Second Decade: Comparison with Unexposed and Non-litigant Groups," *Journal of Applied Social Psychology* 20 (1990): 1,033–1,050.
84. M.C. Grace et al., "The Buffalo Creek Disaster: A 14-Year Follow-Up," in *The International Handbook of Traumatic Stress Syndromes*, eds. J.P. Wilson and B. Raphael (New York: Plenum Press, 1993), 441–449.
85. V.A. Taylor, *Delivery of Mental Health Services in Disasters: The Xenia Tornado and Some Implications* (The Disaster Research Center Book and Monograph Series #11) (Columbus, OH: Disaster Research Center, The Ohio State University, 1976).
86. E.L. Quarantelli, ed., *What Is a Disaster? Perspectives on the Question* (London: Routledge, 1998).
87. B.L. Green and S.D. Solomon, "The Mental Health Impact of Natural and Technological Disasters," in *Traumatic Stress: From Theory to Practice*, eds. J.R. Freedy and S.E. Hobfoll (New York: Plenum Press, 1995), 163–180.
88. R.J. Ursano et al., eds., *Individual and Community Responses to Trauma and Disaster: The Structure of Human Chaos* (Cambridge, England: Cambridge University Press, 1994).
89. K. Erikson, *A New Species of Trouble: The Human Experience of Modern Disasters* (New York: W.W. Norton, 1995).
90. L. Weisaeth, "Psychological and Psychiatric Aspects of Technological Disasters," in *Individual and Community Responses to Trauma and Disaster: The Structure of Human Chaos*, eds. R.J. Ursano et al. (Cambridge, England: Cambridge University Press, 1994), 72–102.
91. J. Kliman et al., "Natural and Human-Made Disasters: Some Therapeutic and Epidemiological Implications for Crisis Intervention," in *Therapeutic Intervention: Healing Strategies for Human Systems*, eds. U. Reuveni et al. (New York: Hu-

man Sciences Press, 1982), 253–280.
92. E.L. Quarantelli, "The Environmental Disasters of the Future Will Be More and Worse But the Prospect Is Not Hopeless," *Disaster Prevention and Management* 2 (1993): 11–25.
93. S.R. Lillibridge, "Industrial Disasters," in *The Public Health Consequences of Disasters*, ed. E.K. Noji (New York: Oxford University Press, 1997), 354–372.
94. International Federation of the Red Cross, "Annex III: The Role of the Red Cross and Red Crescent Societies in Response to Technological Disasters," *International Review of the Red Cross* 310 (1996): 55–130.
95. International Atomic Energy Agency/European Community/World Health Organization, *International Conference: One Decade after Chernobyl: Summing Up the Consequences of the Accident. Summary of the Conference Results, 8–12 April, 1996* (Vienna: 1996).
96. World Health Organization, *Health Consequences of the Chernobyl Accident: Results of the IPHECA Pilot Projects and Related National Programs. Summary Report* (Geneva, Switzerland: 1995).
97. Nuclear Energy Agency, *Chernobyl Ten Years On: Radiological and Health Impact: An Assessment by the NEA Committee on Radiation Protection and Public Health, November 1995* (Paris, France: Organisation for Economic Cooperation and Development Nuclear Energy Agency, 1995).
98. P. Shrivastava, "Long-Term Recovery from the Bhopal Crisis," in *The Long Road to Recovery: Community Responses to Industrial Disaster*, ed. J.K. Mitchell (Tokyo: United Nations University Press, 1996), 121–147.
99. C.E. Fritz, *Disasters and Mental Health: Therapeutic Principles Drawn from Disaster Studies* (Historical and Comparative Disaster Series #10) (Newark, DE: Disaster Research Center, University of Delaware, 1996).
100. B.H. Cuthbertson and J.M. Nigg, "Technological Disaster and the Nontherapeutic Community: A Question of True Victimization," *Environment and Behavior* 19 (1987): 462–483.
101. J.S. Kroll-Smith and S.R. Couch, "Technological Hazards: Social Responses as Traumatic Stressors," in *The International Handbook of Traumatic Stress Syndromes*, eds. J.P. Wilson and B. Raphael (New York: Plenum Press, 1993), 79–91.
102. M.R. Edelstein and A. Wandersman, "Community Dynamics in Coping with Toxic Contaminants," in *Neighborhood and Community Environments*. Vol. 9, eds. I. Altman and A. Wandersman (New York: Plenum Press, 1987), 69–112.
103. M.R. Edelstein, *Contaminated Communities: The Social and Psychosocial Impacts of Residential Toxic Exposure* (Boulder, CO: Westview, 1988).
104. R.E. Kasperson and J.X. Kasperson, "The Social Amplification and Attenuation of Risk," *The Annals of the American Academy of Political and Social Science* 545 (1996): 95–105.
105. A. Baum et al., "Natural Disaster and Technological Catastrophe," *Environment and Behavior* 15 (1983): 333–354.
106. A. Baum, "Toxins, Technology, Disasters," in *Cataclysms, Crises, and Catastrophes: Psychology in Action*, eds. G.R. VandenBos and B.K. Bryant (Washington, DC: American Psychological Association, 1987), 9–53.
107. E.J. Bromet et al., "Long-Term Mental Health Consequences of the Accident at Three Mile Island," *International Journal of Mental Health* 19 (1990): 48–60.
108. J.M. Havenaar et al., "Long-Term Mental Health Effects of the Chernobyl Disaster: An Epidemiologic Survey of Two Former Soviet Regions," *American Journal of Psychiatry* 154 (1997): 1,605–1,607.
109. S.M. Becker, "Psychosocial Assistance after Environmental Accidents: A Policy Perspective," *Environmental Health Perspectives 105,* no. S6 (1997): 1,557–1,563.
110. *Field Manual for Human Service Workers in Major Disasters* (Rockville, MD: National Institute of Mental Health, 1990).
111. S.D. Solomon, "Mobilizing Social Support Networks in Times of Disaster," in *Trauma and Its Wake: Traumatic Stress Theory, Research, and Intervention*, ed. C.R. Figley (New York: Brunner/Mazel Publishers, 1986), 232–263.
112. L.C. Leviton et al., *Confronting Public Health Risks: A Decision Maker's Guide* (Thousand Oaks, CA: Sage Publications, 1998).
113. N.L. Farberow and N.S. Gordon, *Manual for Child Health Workers in Major Disasters* (Washington, DC: Center for Mental Health Services, Substance Abuse and Mental Health Services Administration, U.S. Public Health Service, 1995).
114. L.C. Terr, "Large-Group Preventive Techniques for Use after Disaster," in *Responding to Disaster: A Guide for Mental Health Professionals*, ed. L.S. Austin (Washington, DC: American Psychiatric Press, 1992), 81–99.
115. L.T. Mega and S.L. McCammon, "Tornado in Eastern North Carolina: Outreach to School and Community," in *Responding to Disaster: A Guide for Mental Health Professionals*, ed. L.S. Austin (Washington, DC: American Psychiatric Press, 1992), 211–230.
116. R.S. Pynoos et al., "A Public Mental Health Approach to the Postdisaster Treatment of Children and Adolescents," *Child and Adolescent Psychiatric Clinics of North America* 7 (1988): 195–210.
117. *Responding to the Needs of People with Serious and Persistent Mental Illness in Times of Disaster* (Washington, DC: Emergency Services and Disaster Relief Branch, Center for Mental Health Services, Substance Abuse and Mental Health Services Administration, 1996).
118. American Red Cross Disaster Mental Health Services, *Coping with Disaster: Emotional Health Issues for Disaster Workers on Assignment* (ARC 4472) (Washington, DC: American Red Cross, 1991).
119. American Red Cross Disaster Mental Health Services, *Coping with Disaster: Emotional Health Issues for Families of Disaster Workers* (ARC 4474) (Washington, DC: American Red Cross, 1991).
120. American Red Cross Disaster Mental Health Services, *Coping with Disaster: Returning Home from a Disaster Assignment* (ARC 4473) (Washington, DC: American Red Cross, 1991).
121. J.T. Mitchell and G.S. Everly, Jr., *Critical Incident Stress Debriefing: An Operations Manual for the Prevention of Traumatic Stress among Emergency Service and Disaster Workers,* 2d ed., rev. (Ellicott City, MD: Chevron Publishing Corp., 1997).

122. G.S. Everly, Jr. and J.T. Mitchell, *Critical Incident Stress Management: A New Era and Standard of Care in Crisis Intervention* (Ellicott City, MD: Chevron Publishing Corp., 1997).
123. B. Raphael and J.P. Wilson, "Theoretical and Intervention Considerations in Working with Victims of Disaster," in *International Handbook of Traumatic Stress Syndromes*, eds. J.P. Wilson and B. Raphael (New York: Plenum Press, 1993).
124. J.L. McKnight and J.P. Kretzmann, *Mapping Community Capacity* (Evanston, IL: Center for Urban Affairs and Policy Research, Northwestern University, 1990).
125. N. Bracht, ed., *Health Promotion at the Community Level* (Newbury Park, CA: Sage Publications, 1990).
126. M.V. Melosi, *Pollution and Reform in American Cities, 1870–1930* (Austin, TX: University of Texas Press, 1980).
127. G. Rosen, *A History of Public Health* (Baltimore: Johns Hopkins University Press, 1993).
128. A.E. Peterson et al., "Soap Use Effect on Diarrhea: Nyamithuthu Refugee Camp," *International Journal of Epidemiology* 27 (1998): 520–524.
129. S. Esrey et al., "Effects of Improved Water Supply and Sanitation on Ascariasis, Diarrhoea, Dracunculiasis, Hookworm Infection, Schistosomiasis, and Trachoma," *Bulletin of the World Health Organization 69*, no. 5 (1991): 609–621.
130. "Mortality among Newly Arrived Mozambican Refugees–Zimbabwe and Malawi," *Morbidity and Mortality Weekly Report 42*, no. 24 (1992): 468–477.
131. D. Hatch et al., "Epidemic Cholera during Refugee Resettlement in Malawi," *International Journal of Epidemiology 22*, no. 6 (1994): 1,292–1,299.
132. L.D. Rotz et al., "Bioterrorism Preparedness: Planning for the Future," *Journal of Public Health Management and Practice 6*, no. 4 (2000): 45–49.
133. E. Hood, "Chemical and Biological Weapons: New Questions, New Answers," *Environmental Health Perspectives 107*, no. 12 (1999): 931–932.
134. T. Okumura et al., "The Tokyo Subway Sarin Attack: Disaster Management, Part I: Community Emergency Response," *Academy of Emergency Medicine 5*, no. 6 (1998): 613–617.
135. *The Defense against Weapons of Mass Destruction Act*, The National Defense Authorization Act for Fiscal Year 1997. Title XIV of PL (1996): 104–201.
136. T.J. Cieslak and E.M. Eitzen, "Bioterrorism: Agents of Concern," *Journal of Public Health Management and Practice 6*, no. 4 (2000): 19–29.
137. C.D. Malloy, "A History of Biological and Chemical Warfare and Terrorism," *Journal of Public Health Management and Practice 6*, no. 4 (2000): 30–37.
138. J.A. Popuard and L.A. Miller, "History of Biological Warfare: Catapults to Capsomeres," *Ann NY Acad Sci*, 666 (1992): 9–20.
139. K.B. Olson and Aum Shirikyo, "Once and Future Threat?" *Emerg Inf Dis*, 4 (1999): 513–516.
140. L.A. Cole, "Bioterrorism Threats: Learning from Inappropriate Responses," *Journal of Public Health Management and Practice 6*, no. 4 (2000): 8–18.
141. U.S. Centers for Disease Control and Prevention, "Bioterrorism Alleging Use of Anthrax and Interim Guidelines for Management," *1998 MMWR Weekly Review 48*, no. 4 (1999): 69–74.
142. L.C. Garrett et al., "Taking the Terror Out of Bioterrorism: Planning for a Bioterrorist Event from a Local Perspective," *Journal of Public Health Management and Practice 6*, no. 4 (2000): 1–7.
143. U.S. Centers for Disease Control and Prevention, National Center for Infectious Diseases, *Critical Agents of Concern, Summary of Selection Process and Recommendations* (Atlanta, GA: publisher, 1999).
144. Cohen et al. "Bioterrorism Initiatives: Public Health in Reverse?" *American Journal of Public Health 84*, no. 11 (1999): 1,629–1,631.

Taking the Terror Out of Bioterrorism: Planning for a Bioterrorist Event from a Local Perspective

Larry C. Garrett, Charles Magruder, and Craig A. Molgard

There is a growing concern in the public health community over the potential for domestic biological and chemical acts of terrorism. These types of events do not respect city limits, county lines, or other geopolitical borders and pose a unique challenge for local health departments that have a critical role in detecting, preparing for, and responding to such events. Because direct support for most public health service, including bioterrorism preparedness, occurs primarily at the local level, this is the logical starting point for all planning activities.

Introduction

There is a growing concern in the public health community over the potential for domestic biological and chemical acts of terrorism. These types of events do not respect city limits, county lines, or other geopolitical borders and pose a unique challenge for local health departments that have a critical role in detecting, preparing for, and responding to such events.[1]

The bombing of the World Trade Center in New York City and the Alfred P. Murrah Federal Building in Oklahoma City have forced Americans to face the reality that terrorism is not something that occurs only overseas. According to U.S. intelligence agencies, conventional explosives continue to be the weapon of choice for terrorists, while chemical and biological materials are less likely to be used because they are more difficult to weaponize and the results are unpredictable.[2] However, nations and dissident groups exist that have both the motivation and access to skills to selectively cultivate some of the most dangerous pathogens and to deploy them as agents of terrorism or war.[3]

There have already been several troubling incidents. In 1984, for example, 751 people became ill after two members of an Oregon sect produced and

Larry C. Garrett, MPH, *is an Epidemiologist with the Centers for Disease Control and Prevention in Atlanta, Georgia.*

Charles Magruder, MD, MPH, *is Director of the Wichita Sedgwick County Department of Community Health in Wichita, Kansas.*

Craig A. Molgard, PhD, MPH, *is a Professor and Director of the Master of Public Health Program, Department of Preventive Medicine, University of Kansas School of Medicine in Wichita, Kansas.*

distributed Salmonella, an intestinal organism, in restaurants to affect the outcome of a local election. One year later, four members of an anti-government militia group were convicted of planning to use ricin to kill government workers. Ricin, one of the most poisonous substances known to man, is derived from the common castor bean. Also in 1995, the Japanese cult, Aum Shinrikyo, released the nerve agent Sarin in the Tokyo subway and had plans for biological terrorism; included in its arsenal were botulinum toxin and anthrax cultures. In November 1995, an alleged member of a white supremacist group pled guilty to possession of three vials of Yersinia pestis, the organism that is capable of causing bubonic, septicemic, and pneumonic plague. In December 1998, the Federal Bureau of Investigation (FBI) and U.S. Army biological warfare experts raided a farm in Arkansas and found 130 grams of ricin, enough to kill 30,000 people if properly dispensed.[4]

This article summarizes the events surrounding the alleged threat of anthrax in a local office building in Wichita, Kansas, in August 1998. In addition, the authors review the response of the local health department and apply the lessons learned from this incident to bioterrorism preparedness activities. It must be noted that because this case is still under criminal investigation, the authors did not have complete access to all of the official data and timelines, making some of the information presented subject to change.

Background

On August 18, 1998, several hundred workers were evacuated and a four-block area of downtown Wichita was cordoned off after a suspicious white powder was found in an office building. The evacuation began around 11:00 AM when the substance was found spread on several stairwells and elevators in the building. The office for Social and Rehabilitation Services, one of the many government agencies housed in the building, had received a threatening letter in a manila envelope stating the substance was anthrax.

Local emergency medical services (EMS), hazardous material units (HAZMAT), health department, and law enforcement officials detained nearly 200 people who may have been exposed; all persons in the area where the white powder was found and in the office that had received the letter were considered possibly exposed to *Bacillus anthracis* spores. Overall control of the operation was directed by the FBI, with support from the Department of Defense (DoD) because the two are lead agencies involving biological acts or threats of terrorism. Because the local authorities had limited expertise with biological threats, the DoD assumed the primary role in the sampling and identification of the substance at the scene.

HAZMAT personnel responded in full protective gear with self-contained respirators to assess and contain the area. The air-handling system in the building was turned off to reduce the potential spread of *Bacillus anthracis* spores. Evacuation of the building was completed and the detained individuals were placed on air-conditioned buses near the building to ensure their comfort and keep them at the scene while the validity of the threat was assessed. The desktop where the letter was opened was washed with a 5 percent hypochlorite solution after collection of evidence by the FBI.

Five hours after the substance was found, most of the detained individuals were allowed to leave. This decision was made following a conference call coordinated by the FBI in which experts determined that it was very unlikely the substance was *Bacillus anthracis* due to its physical properties and lack of an effective dispersal method. The contributors to this decision included specialists from the Centers for Disease Control and Prevention (CDC), the DoD, and the Kansas Department of Health and Environment (KDHE). Before departing, contact information for follow-up was collected by public health officials and arrangements were made for counseling. Each person received detailed instructions to shower and double bag their clothes in plastic when they returned home. A handful of people who came in direct contact with the substance were decontaminated in a temporary shelter provided by McConnell Air Force base using soap, water, and a dilute bleach solution.

The DoD completed the on-site testing of the alleged *Bacillus anthracis* using an Enzyme Immuno Assay testing procedure (similar to a rapid strep test) known as a "Smart Card." The definitive testing of the substance was conducted by the United States Army Research Institute for Infectious Diseases, DoD, in Fort Detrick, Maryland where direct fluorescent antibody testing and culture were negative.

Within 24 hours after the initial threat, lab results showed the substance posed no chemical or biological threat.

Health Department Response

Immediately after the EMS and law enforcement officials were notified of the potential anthrax exposure, a health department environmental health staff member trained for HAZMAT response was called to the scene. Due to the large public health consequences of anthrax, the city manager directly contacted the director of the health department and requested that he personally respond. The director of environmental health and a nurse epidemiologist also reported to the scene. They were equipped with two-way radios and a cellular telephone enabling them to maintain contact with the health department for ongoing support and access to additional sources of information as needed. Health department staff gathered information on *Bacillus anthracis* and its health consequences via exposure through inhalation and established contact with the CDC's Emergency Response Center and KDHE's Office of Epidemiological Services.

The health department's nurse epidemiologist collected contact information for follow-up, including name, address, phone number, location in building, time in/out of the building, and if visiting the building, whom the person saw. This information was gathered to help the health department if it became necessary to treat this population prophylactically. Instructions were given to the potentially exposed individuals on the need to shower and the proper handling of personal belongings until the substance had been identified. The director of the health department requested a mental health team to come to the scene to provide needed support, particularly for those who could not return home immediately and had to go through the decontamination process.

At the health department, work was underway to find a source of appropriate antibiotics and anthrax vaccine. In addition, the staff was preparing for the delivery of the pharmaceuticals if the substance was found to be *Bacillus anthracis*. Contact was maintained with the CDC's Emergency Response Center and information was relayed to and from the scene via telephone and radio. The health department staff maintained a "cautionary vigilant" stance until the substance was identified positively as a non-threat. The final role played by the health department was to provide notification to the exposed individuals that they were indeed safe and that the substance they were exposed to was of no threat.

Lessons Learned

Many important issues became readily apparent pertaining to the health department's emergency response procedures. These included weaknesses with communication, lack of a functional information management system, and inadequate training for bioterrorism response.

Communication

Communication became an immediate problem between health department personnel at the scene and support staff at the health department. The use of radios was difficult at times and not always accomplished. In addition, communication over open airwaves was not secure, making confidential discussion impossible. Further, the cellular telephone did not work adequately due to location and limited battery life. Part of the communication problem was due to the county not fully activating its Emergency Operations Center. This type of event was unforeseen in the county's Emergency Response Plan and resulted in a failure for the county to follow portions of its basic emergency protocol; this is an area that is being evaluated at this time.

Information systems

The lack of access to an effective and flexible information system hindered the collection of the facts necessary to support the health department's operations. Up-to-date information on bioterrorism and anthrax became problematic as Internet resources at the health department were limited to only one computer. In addition, there was no previous planning or training that had taken place at the health department concerning bioterrorism.

Other difficulties related to the lack of a flexible surveillance system. Currently, the health department relies on a statewide computer-based disease surveillance system. This system lacks flexibility and will not adapt to an event-driven incident and the individuals associated with it. In addition, the nurse epidemiologist was not familiar with standard

CDC epidemiology programs (i.e., Epi-Info), making the use of computerized data collection impossible. This resulted in health department personnel using a paper-based system to collect relevant data and the double entry of the data before letters could be sent notifying the affected individuals that the substance they were exposed to posed no threat.

More importantly, a review of the data collected after the event revealed that core information such as phone numbers or addresses was missing, making contact with a significant proportion of this population virtually impossible. Problems such as these have potentially life-threatening consequences.

Training in bioterrorism response

A review of the county's and health department's Emergency Response Plans revealed there were no written plans or guidelines to respond to biological threats; this may have slowed notification of the proper authorities and perhaps delayed the actual identification of the unknown substance. The lack of specific training and preparation caused other problems as well, including the health department's environmental health responder with the HAZMAT crews not notifying the director of the health department of the potential public health disaster; having both the health department director and the director of environmental health at the scene simultaneously; and lack of a central point of control for all health department activities, including the management of incoming and outgoing information. A written response plan that all staff had reviewed and practiced in mock disaster drills beforehand would have removed some uncertainty surrounding the event.

Discussion

The majority of health departments across the U.S. do not have a plan to respond to a biological attack. Because terrorists are opportunists by nature, as a nation, we are vulnerable to an attack. The potential spectrum of bioterrorism ranges from hoaxes to state-sponsored terrorism that employs classic biological warfare techniques designed to produce mass casualties.[5] Of particular concern are smallpox, anthrax, and plague.[6] The planning to meet these threats needs to start at the community level as local health departments are the first line of defense; too often, planning at the state and federal level neglects this important concept.

Local level capacity

In 1995, the National Association of County and City Health Officials (NACCHO) conducted a capacity assessment of local health departments throughout the nation. The study found that most local health departments are small and rely on limited staff, information systems, and financial resources. In addition, they found that there are serious deficiencies affecting the ability of local health departments to respond to public health emergencies. Moreover, local health department workers represent a wide range of occupations, including nurses, nurse practitioners, physician assistants, sanitation workers, and environmental health specialists.[7] There was a noted lack of trained epidemiologists and other public health professionals; these professionals are necessary to direct core public health activities including disease surveillance, communicable/infectious disease control, and other public health activities. These shortcomings create a risk for the entire nation, not simply selected cities or localities, especially when confronting bioterrorism events.

CDC funding

The CDC announced the availability of 40 million dollars in fiscal year 1999 to enhance public health preparedness and response for bioterrorism. A large portion of this cooperative funding agreement is to be used to develop local capacity. Specific areas of focus include preparedness planning and readiness assessment; expansion of surveillance and epidemiology capacity; increased laboratory capacity for chemical/biological agent identification; and the development of effective communication linkages and public health training capacity.

Response strategies to bioterrorism

When planning a response strategy to bioterrorism, local health departments should identify key responders within their jurisdiction including EMS, law enforcement, and emergency management agencies. Defining the roles of each agency, including protection of first responders, is important.[8] Many of these agencies may already be working on their own programs and integrating the public health response within their plans may be an effective use of resources. Health department directors should familiarize themselves with the Nunn-Lugar-Domenici Act of 1997, which provides funding and federal support to enhance community response capability to biological and chemical events. Health officers also need to familiarize themselves with their local and state public health status and regulations, particularly those concerning isolation and quarantine of persons afflicted with infectious or contagious disease. The development of fact sheets on the most common biological and chemical threats should be considered for distribution to local medical providers to help them recognize the signs and symptoms of biological/chemical agents for inclusion in their differential diagnosis. The training of likely first responders (i.e., emergency department physicians) needs to be part of a comprehensive readiness plan.

Casualties and capabilities

With few exceptions, treatment of a small number of individuals exposed to a chemical or biological agent is not beyond current medical capabilities; however, large numbers of casualties would overtax those capabilities quickly. Planning should include methods to enhance decontamination capabilities and supplementation of medical providers with personnel trained to respond to biological or chemical events. Assessment of local area hospitals on supplies of antidotes, drugs, ventilators, personal protective equipment, decontamination capacity, mass-casualty planning and training, isolation rooms for infectious disease, and familiarity of staff with the effects and treatment of chemical and biological weapons[9] are additional assessment and planning activities that must be conducted locally.

Disease surveillance at the local level

Expanding disease surveillance and epidemiological capacity at the local level is an important component of bioterrorism preparedness. Not all acts of bioterrorism will be large-scale events and may involve only a small portion of a targeted population. This could be accomplished by dispersing pathogens in enclosed spaces or poisoning pharmaceuticals, prepared food, livestock, or crops. These types of situations may be missed or dismissed as background noise on a large state-based disease surveillance system but may be captured on a local one. For example, nearly all of the investigations that lead to the recognition of infectious disease outbreaks throughout the United States are initiated by local health departments,[1] and a local nurse or epidemiologist may be the first to identify a potential bioterrorism event through routine local disease surveillance activities; this is especially true if the pathogen is a "nontraditional" biological warfare agent (e.g., Salmonella). Local disease surveillance is an essential first step in preparedness and is important in helping law enforcement officials to react swiftly.[5]

Types of incident categories

Surveillance systems at the local level must be able to capture and support three types of incident categories: (1) event driven, (2) disease specific, and (3) total counts. A bioterrorist or chemical incident is event driven and the surveillance system must be able to accommodate one to many individuals associated with the event; basic identification, demographic, and exposure data should be collected. A disease-specific event is where an individual is associated with a specific disease; this is the traditional model of reportable disease surveillance. Total count is the ability to aggregate numbers of specific diseases without the need to capture personal identifiers or demographic data; total cases of gastroenteritis in a school district are an example of this type of capacity.

"Buy in" from locals

The analysis of surveillance data is, in principle, quite simple. Data are examined by measures of time, place, and person.[10] Surveillance systems at the local level do not have to be elaborate to meet these needs, but they must be inclusive. It is important to seek "buy in" from local hospitals, clinics, and other health care providers in the local area as they are the providers of data. If a state is using an electronic disease surveillance system, efforts must be made to integrate the local system with the state system to facilitate bi-directional flow of data without the need to reenter data. By strengthening local surveillance capacity, the overall capacity of the state increases as well. Multiple points of entry into the surveillance system are important, and the development of electronic data capture while simultaneously accepting telephone and paper reports should be encouraged. It is important to provide feedback to the providers of surveillance data in the form of reports, updates, and other pertinent information. This will help assure them that the data are used for appropriate public health surveillance activities.

Developing local capacity

Developing local epidemiological capacity is vital for increased bioterrorism preparedness. There are many ways to increase this capacity, including the use of distance learning programs provided by the CDC and a variety of summer and special training programs offered by universities and schools of public health around the country. The merits of updating a surveillance system without having staff trained with basic epidemiological skills should be considered carefully.

Identification of support laboratories

While the expansion of laboratory capacity for the identification of chemical and biological agents is vital to the overall success of bioterrorism preparedness, generally it is beyond the scope of all but the largest health departments and therefore should be a state-based activity. However, local health departments need to be aware of their state's capacity and be able to identify the nearest laboratory to be used for biological and chemical identification. In some instances, particularly for potential biological material, capacity may be limited to a handful of labs in the entire country.

Modern systems and skills

To address bioterrorism threats effectively, local health departments must be given modern information systems and staff equipped with advanced, regularly updated professional skills. Unfortunately, most local health departments are forced to rely on outdated communication and information systems and many of their workers lack access to required training. A 1996 study conducted by NACCHO[11] revealed that many health departments have no access to the Internet or other essential on-line data and communication services; one-half of all local health departments did not use electronic mail (e-mail); computers are scarce commodities for many health workers and staff in 70 percent of the departments had "little or no expertise" in using on-line health data and services available from the CDC, state health departments, and other authoritative sources.

As local health departments attempt to overcome their lack of computer and telecommunications infrastructure, the initial challenge facing them will be how to transcend the surface appeal of computer technology and harness its power to improve the health of populations. Simply building an e-mail system with access to the Internet is not sufficient. Serious consideration needs to be given to systems integration. Traditionally, integration efforts have been attempted at the state or regional level and most ran out of resources before reaching the operational stage.

Because direct support for most public health service—including bioterrorism preparedness—occurs primarily at the local level, this is the logical starting point for all integration activities. However, this approach is nontraditional, may face "political" opposition, and will take several years to plan, develop, and implement. Because not all health departments have large staff or resources, grouping together and sharing scarce resources, expertise, and services may help ease the development of integrated public health information systems. These groupings also may help in the development of effective bioterrorism response plans. Many local health departments do not have the staff or expertise to develop their own plan while a regional grouping of health departments can share resources and responsibilities and can form synergistic relationships that will benefit the entire public health community.

■ ■ ■

Given the current state of biological and chemical bioterrorism preparedness at local health departments throughout the country, the staff at the Wichita-Sedgwick Department of Community Health did an excellent job. Their action and flexibility represent the true spirit of public health and dedication to protecting the health of the community. The alleged use of *Bacillus anthracis* in Wichita should be used as an opportunity to assess local public health officials' actions and strengthen their response, for they may not be as fortunate in the future. Preparation and an increase in the capacity of local health departments are the keys to ensure an organized and successful response to this sinister public health threat.

REFERENCES

1. Centers for Disease Control and Prevention, *Strengthening Community Health Protection through Technology and Training: The Health Alert Network.* Atlanta, GA: Centers for Disease Control and Prevention, 1998.
2. United States General Accounting Office, *Combating Terrorism: Federal Agencies' Efforts to Implement National Policy and Strategy*. GAO Pub. No. GAO/NSIAD–97–254. Washington, DC: U.S. Government Printing Office, 1997.
3. D.A. Henderson, "Bioterrorism as a Public Health Threat," *Emerging Infectious Diseases* 4, no. 3 (July–Sept 1998).
4. S.F. Tomajczyk, "Preparing for the Ultimate Public Health Nightmare," *The American Journal of Health Communications* 2, no. 1 (1997): 5–11.
5. J.E. McDade and D. Franz, "Bioterrorism as a Public Health Threat," *Emerging Infectious Diseases* 4, no. 3 (July Sept 1998).
6. A. Vorobyov, *Criterion Rating as a Measure of Probable Use of Bioagents as Biological Weapons.* Paper presented to the Working Group on Biological Weapons Control of the Committee on International Security and Arms Control, National Academy of Sciences, Washington, DC, April 1994.
7. National Association of County and City Health Officials. *1992–1993 National Profile of Local Health Departments.* Washington, DC: National Association of County and City Health Officials, 1995.
8. Centers for Disease Control and Prevention, "Bioterrorism Alleging Use of Anthrax and Interim Guidelines for Management—United States, 1998," *Morbidity and Mortality Weekly Report* 48, no. 4 (1999): 69–74.
9. Institute of Medicine, *Improving Civilian Response to Chemical or Biological Terrorist Incidents: Interim Report on Current Capabilities.* Washington, DC: National Academy Press, 1998.
10. S.M. Teutsch and R.E. Churchill, eds., *Principles and Practice of Public Health Surveillance.* New York: Oxford University Press, 1994.
11. National Association of County and City Health Officials, *Study of Electronic Communication Capacity of Local Health Departments.* Washington, DC: National Association of County and City Health Officials, 1996.

Bioterrorism Threats: Learning from Inappropriate Responses

Leonard A. Cole

Between April 1997 and June 1999, some 200 mailed or telephoned bioterrorism threats were received at a variety of locations. Usually claiming that anthrax had been released, the threats all proved to be hoaxes. In many instances, local emergency responders treated the more than 13,000 potential victims inappropriately, in particular requiring victims to strip and undergo decontamination with bleach solutions. Narratives of several incidents indicated that many victims were distressed and embarrassed by their treatment. Their experiences underscore the need for improved local response actions and the formulation of a uniform response protocol for public health agencies.

INTELLIGENCE AND PUBLIC health experts believe that the threat of bioterrorism has grown sharply in recent years.[1,2] Their concerns have been widely reported in the media along with dramatic warnings by government leaders about the effects of biological weapons.[3] Anthrax in particular has been prominently publicized as a likely biological weapon.[4] One disquieting byproduct of the publicity has been a rash of bioterrorism scares, usually involving a claim that people have been exposed to anthrax.[5] All the alarms proved to be false, but the stunning increase in their number through mid-1999 was underscored at a congressional hearing. An official from the Federal Bureau of Investigation (FBI) testified that in 1997, the bureau had logged 27 bioterrorism threats; in 1998, the figure was 112 and in the first half of 1999, it had exceeded 100.[6]

A report by the Centers for Disease Control and Prevention (CDC) in February 1999 reviewed seven bioterrorism threats that occurred toward the end of 1998.[7] As with most such incidents, they involved letters claiming that the reader had been exposed to anthrax or telephone calls claiming the bacteria were in ventilation systems. Protective measures employed by emergency responders (police, firefighters, paramedics) varied. At some locations, the presumed victims were told to go home, place their clothes in plastic bags, and shower. At others, they were quarantined, made to disrobe and undergo scrubbing with diluted bleach, and begin taking antibiotics. In a few cases, victims were hospitalized. In each case, after a day or two—or sometimes longer—laboratory tests showed no evidence of anthrax contamination.

Inconsistent responses arose in part from unclear or contradictory guidelines from different agencies.

***Leonard A. Cole, PhD,** is a Political Science Professor at Rutgers University in Newark, New Jersey.*

A 1998 Anthrax Advisory by the FBI, for example, said that if "there is confirmation" of anthrax exposure, victims should undergo decontamination with a diluted household bleach solution, specifically "Clorox—5.25% hypochlorite."[8] When confronted with an actual threat, many local authorities ignored the requirement to confirm the presence of anthrax. Acting on the side of caution, they required potential victims to be scrubbed anyway. The CDC's February 1999 report advised that presumed victims be washed with soap and water, but also suggested decontaminating "the environment in direct contact with [a possibly contaminated] letter or its contents . . . with a 0.5% hypochlorite solution (i.e., one part household bleach to 10 parts water)."[7] Whether or not the "environment" included the people who had been in direct contact was not made clear. A June 1999 document prepared by the Association for Professionals in Infection Control and Epidemiology (APIC) in cooperation with the CDC was more definitive: "Decontamination should only be considered in instances of gross contamination." In bold print, the document also stated: "Potentially harmful practices, such as bathing patients with bleach solutions, are unnecessary and should be avoided."[9] The APIC statement apparently was the first that explicitly warned against washing people with bleach because it could cause them harm. Moreover, it was followed in August with an observation by CDC officials that "the actual efficacy of disinfection with sodium hypochlorite in cases of bioterrorism is questionable."[10]

Scrubbing victims with bleach solutions was not the only questionable practice exhibited by emergency responders to bioterrorism threats. Many incidents in the past two years involved other erratic actions as well. Inconsistencies may be seen in Table 1, which lists information on 40 anthrax hoaxes. Representing about 20 percent of the total of some 200 incidents that occurred between April 1997 and June 1999, they were selected because of either of two criteria: (1) available information indicated large numbers of people were affected or (2) aggressive treatments were rendered. Although drawn largely from news articles, data were augmented by official reports and interviews by the author with officials and victims.

Actual numbers of evacuated or quarantined victims were available only for 30 of the 40 listed incidents. These totaled 12,398. The numbers reported for the 10 other listed incidents were variously described as "several" or "hundreds." Thus, for the 40 incidents, the number of lives disrupted approached 13,000. For the approximate 200 incidents, the figure almost surely far exceeded 13,000.

Among the 40 listed hoaxes, in 26 of them, victims underwent decontamination (usually with bleach solution), and in 20, they received antibiotic treatment and/or were hospitalized. In 30 of the incidents (75 percent of the total), potential victims were subjected to at least one of these aggressive responses. The figures doubtless represent higher proportions of these responses than occurred among all the bioterrorism threats. For many of the unlisted incidents, details were unavailable. But based on probability, several of the unlisted incidents also likely involved large numbers of victims and aggressive emergency responses.

Table 1 reveals the breadth of inconsistency but nothing about psychological effects on victims. Interviews indicated that several people in the targeted areas were unfazed and considered the episodes minor inconveniences. But many were terrified. Similarly, some felt that emergency response teams acted efficiently and sensitively. Others, even months after their experiences, were bitter about having undergone embarrassing and intrusive treatment.

By mid-1999, despite the introduction of more clear and rational protocols, response skills at the local level remained uncertain. Moreover, an important area still receiving little attention was the attitudes of the presumed victims. Descriptions of several incidents demonstrate the variety of responses and their effects on the victims.

B'nai B'rith, Washington, DC, April 1997

The first large-scale anthrax hoax occurred on April 24, 1997, at the Washington, DC offices of B'nai B'rith, an international Jewish service organization. At 11:30 AM, a mail room employee noticed a foul-smelling package that was leaking a red gelatinous substance.[11,12] He brought the parcel to the organization's director of security, Carmen Fontana, who called the police. "We were thinking 'bomb,'" Fontana recalled. (Personal communication, June 7, 1999.) When the police opened the package, they found a petri dish containing a material labeled "anthrachs," according to news reports.[11] (A report

Table 1

Forty selected anthrax hoaxes, April 1997–June 1999 (based on whether victims were reported to have received treatment or if large numbers were affected)

Date	Location	Target	Threat communication	Threat material or technique	Evacuated or quarantined (approx)	Decontam-inated (some or all)	Hospital and/or antibiotics (some or all)
6–15–99	Hempstead, NY	courthouse	letter	brown stain	500		
6–15–99	Mineola, NY	courthouse	letter	brown stain	500		
5–17–99	Syracuse, NY	college (Catholic)	letter	white powder	30	yes	yes
4–22–99	Kansas City, MO	IRS offices	letter*	dark substance	2,000	yes	
4–19–99	Biloxi, MS	courthouse	note	ventilation system	100		
3–3–99	Salt Lake City, UT	church	package and note	contents of package	several	yes	yes
2–26–99	Boise, ID	Planned Parenthood	letter	powder	24	yes	yes
2–24–99	Salt Lake City, UT	Planned Parenthood	package and note	contents of package	20	yes	yes
2–23–99	Pittsburgh, PA	abortion clinic	letter	contents	3+	yes	
2–22–99	St. Louis, MO	Planned Parenthood	letter	contents	several	yes	
2–22–99	Kansas City, MO	Planned Parenthood	letter	dark smudge	27	yes	yes
2–22–99	New York City, NY	Planned Parenthood	letter	contents	several		
2–18–99	Milwaukee, WI	Womens Health Org.	package and letter	smudge	hundreds	yes	yes
2–18–99	Cincinnati, OH	abortion clinic	package and letter	contents	4	yes	yes
2–18–99	Manchester, NH	Planned Parenthood	package and letter	white powder	several	yes	
2–18–99	Spokane County, OR	Planned Parenthood	letter	contents	3+	yes	
2–12–99	Los Angeles, CA	*LA Times* Building	letter	gray powder	2,000		
2–4–99	Atlanta, GA	NBC news office	package and letter	black powder	600	yes	yes
2–4–99	Washington, DC	*Washington Post*	letter	contents	several	yes	
2–2–99	Lackawanna, NY	high school and library	phone	spread in buildings	several		
1–13–99	Tualatin, OR	library and city offices	phone	spread in buildings	several		
1–2–99	Anaheim, CA	high school	phone	ventilation system	120		
12–31–98	Rochester, NY	federal building	letter	contents	1+	yes	yes

continues

Table 1
Continued

Date	Location	Target	Threat communication	Threat material or technique	Evacuated or quarantined (approx)	Decontam-inated (some or all)	Hospital and/or antibiotics (some or all)
12–26–98	Pomona, CA	nightclub	phone	ventilation system	800		
12–24–98	Palm Desert, CA	department store	phone	ventilation system	200	yes	
12–23–98	Chatsworth, CA	cable TV company	phone	unspecified	200	yes	
12–21–98	Van Nuys, CA	two courthouses	phone	ventilation system	2,000		yes
12–18–98	Woodland Hills, CA	courthouse	phone	unspecified	90	yes	yes
12–17–98	Westwood, CA	office building	letter	contents	21	yes	yes
12–4–98	Coppell, TX	post office	vial*	contents	500	yes	
11–18–98	Miami Beach, FL	fashion magazine office	letter	white powder	19	yes	yes
11–10–98	Seymour, IN	Walmart and bank	letter	contents	several		yes
11–10–98	Bloomington, IN	high school	letter	white crystalline material	1,800		
11–9–98	Indianapolis, IN	church and school (Catholic)	letter	brown powder	480	yes	yes
11–9–98	Cheektogawa, NY	church (Catholic)	letter	contents	9	yes	yes
11–2–98	Toledo, OH	abortion clinic	letter	contents	3	yes	yes
10–31–98	Louisville, KY	abortion clinic	letter	brown powder	several		yes
10–30–98	Indianapolis, IN	Planned Parenthood	letter	brown powder	31	yes	yes
8–18–98	Wichita, KS	state office building	note	white powder on stairs and elevators	200		
4–24–97	Washington, DC	B'nai B'rith	mailed petri dish	red gelatinous substance	109+	yes	yes
					12,398 (+10 incidents reporting "several" or "hundreds")	26	20

* Did not name contents, but assumed to be anthrax.

Note: The information in this table is based on news reports and interviews with officials and participants in the incidents. The 40 listed incidents represent about one fifth of the total number of anthrax hoaxes recorded by the FBI during this period.

by the Federal Emergency Management Agency [FEMA] said the dish was labeled "*Anthracis Yersinia.*")[12] The fire department's hazardous materials (HAZMAT) unit was summoned and kept the dozen people who had been near the package in isolation. Upon learning of its presumed contents, Fontana, a 56-year-old retired police officer, recalled that he, like others, assumed the worst: "I was a little nervous when I thought it was a bomb. When I found out it was anthrax and I had taken a deep breath of it, I believed I was dead." (Personal communication, June 7, 1999.)

The fire department sealed off a one-block area surrounding the B'nai B'rith building. The 109 people in the building and an unknown number in a hotel across the street were quarantined.[12] HAZMAT and emergency medical services (EMS) personnel consulted with CDC officials, who advised that the victims be decontaminated with a one-percent bleach solution.[12] Meanwhile, the package had been turned over to the FBI and then delivered for analysis to the National Naval Medical Center in Bethesda, Maryland. A measure of the tension and confusion was captured in a paragraph of the FEMA report.

> Personnel then waited for the results of the testing. During this time, a security guard in the quarantine area developed chest pains. He was carried on a chair through the decontaminated corridor and then transported to a local hospital. . . . Also during this waiting period, several MPD (Metropolitan Police Department) officers became upset with instruction that they undergo decontamination. The officers had become aware that the media was broadcasting live pictures from cameras positioned on top of a nearby building. The officers refused to disrobe and undergo decontamination. One of the officers struck the EMS lieutenant assigned to the quarantine area. High-ranking police officials were asked to help get the officers to comply with the procedures and, eventually, the officers were decontaminated.

The quarantine ended after nine hours when laboratory analysis found no evidence that material in the package was dangerous.

The FEMA report offers a valuable, if limited, review of the incident and the shortcomings of the response procedures. Fontana, the B'nai B'rith's director of security, was more pointed in his assessment of the fire department's HAZMAT and EMS crews. "No one really knew what to do," he said. (Personal communication, June 7, 1999.) According to Fontana, the responders went to a supermarket and bought Clorox bleach off the shelf. They then sprayed it at the 30 naked civilians, police, and fire personnel who had to undergo decontamination. After the spraying, the victims were given coverall suits and escorted to a bus. "We sat on the bus for eight hours, reeking of Clorox," Fontana said. He elaborated on his initial reluctance to obey the directive to go outdoors in front of the building, undress, and be sprayed. "I got into an argument with the fire commander. I told him I did not want my 14-year-old granddaughter to see me stripped down on television." The fire commander said that the decontamination site would be near a fire engine, which would block the view of outsiders. However, television cameras on a nearby rooftop had visual access to the decontamination. Videos of the event, including naked people being sprayed, appeared on the evening news. "Ironically, my granddaughter did see me on TV, stripped. She panicked," Fontana said. Another B'nai B'rith employee was so embarrassed by the ordeal that he never came back to work there again.

The FEMA report notes that the absence of tents for decontamination meant that people had to "disrobe in front of television cameras." As a result of the experience, the report hoped that HAZMAT departments in the future would become better prepared to consider "the public's modesty." It also spoke to the confusion of advice about whether the occupants of the building should have been kept in place and the ventilation system shut down. The report noted that some health professionals thought that approach wrong. "By isolating people in an unventilated and possibly contaminated area, the victims were in effect exposed . . . for an extended duration."[12] Other experts gave contrary advice, based on the notion that when exposed to a biological agent, a person cannot be effectively decontaminated. Therefore, "possible victims should be simply treated, observed, or sent home."[12] The report's concluding observation left the matter in limbo: "More research is needed to address the question of whether it is best to protect in-place or to evacuate to a safe haven, those civilians exposed to chem-bio agents."[12]

In the 18 months after the B'nai B'rith incident, a few other anthrax hoaxes were reported, though the frequency began to accelerate toward the end of 1998. By early 1999, they were averaging at least one a day, according to an FBI spokesman.[13] Still, local responses often remained inappropriate.

NBC News Office, Atlanta, Georgia, February 1999

The NBC network news office in Atlanta is on the 11th floor of a 12-story office building. Around noon on Thursday, February 4, 1999, an NBC employee opened a mailed envelope containing a baggie full of material that looked like dark sand and pepper. An accompanying letter said: "You and everyone in this building have been exposed to anthrax."[14] (Personal communication, NBC staff member who requested not to be identified by name, June 21, 1999.) People in the office called 911, the FBI, and the CDC. Two plainclothes police officers quickly came over from the police headquarters across the street. Later, more emergency responders arrived, including more police and paramedics.

All seven NBC employees and the two plainclothes police officers were sprayed with a bleach solution while in the office and fully dressed. Then, in wet clothing, the nine victims were taken to the elevator and down to the lobby. The lobby was filling with people from other floors who had learned of the anthrax threat and were trying to leave the building. As the nine victims got off the elevator, other police officers ordered them to return upstairs. Meanwhile, officials were sealing off a four-block area.[15] (Personal communication, Lieutenant Reggie Lattimer, Head of Special Operations of the Atlanta Fire Department, July 8, 1999.) Initially, several people were evacuated from the building. Some time later, however, those still inside were prevented from leaving. All told, about 600 people were evacuated or quarantined, according to Lattimer.

Fire department personnel arrived 45 minutes after the first telephone calls. Some were dressed in masks and protective outerwear and went up to the 11th floor, where they sprayed the hallways and the NBC office with a bleach solution. The nine victims also received a second spraying, again while fully dressed.

An NBC staff member recounted her experience. Felice (a pseudonym) was among the nine who were sprayed. Her clothing, like that of the others, had turned pale from the bleach. When interviewed four months after the incident, she noted that the carpeting in the office was still bleached out and no one was sure when it would be replaced. After undergoing the second spraying in the office, the nine were again taken down to the lobby by elevator. This time they were escorted out of the building to awaiting ambulances. Still clothed and drenched, Felice and another woman went into one of the ambulances, but were immediately ordered out because "someone said we might be contaminating the ambulance." (Personal communication, July 8, 1999.)

The two women were taken to a nearby HAZMAT truck where, along with the other victims, they were decontaminated again. One at a time, the nine victims undressed and submitted to a third bleach washdown. Following a shower in the truck with plain water, they were given sheets to wrap themselves in. As they exited the truck, a man held a tarp to block the view of onlookers. There were not enough ambulances for everyone, so the five women were taken to those available while the four men were left to wait until other ambulances arrived. Once in the ambulance, Felice was told she would have to be hooked to an intravenous (IV) line. She objected strenuously. "I hate needles," she said, but was told she had no choice.

Upon arriving at Grady hospital, the victims found that outdoor showers had been set up on a platform in front of the entrance. Felice and the other women were told they could not enter the hospital until taking a shower (their fourth decontamination). "The area was not closed off, and we had to take off our sheets and go under the shower in public view." While still attached to the IV line, Felice washed herself with the detergent soap she was given. "For some of us, the water was so hot it felt scalding. But others had very cold water. It really was erratic." Inside the hospital, the five women were given hospital greens to wear. Soon after, they were told that initial laboratory tests of the threat material showed no evidence of anthrax. The test results became available before the male victims were brought to the hospital so they were spared the shower in public view.

Felice says she felt less troubled by the experience than some of her coworkers. "They were angry they had to go through this," she said. "The thing that mainly got to me personally was having to have the IV. For what purpose?" In the days afterward, Felice thought about the event and how poorly it was handled. She wondered why the men holding the tarps up were not in "moon suits" when all the other personnel were. "That made no sense to me." Also, she said that it was difficult to understand what people were saying while in their masks. Much of the time, the victims tried to interpret hand motions by the personnel in masks because their commands were unintelligible. Moreover, Felice felt frustrated by a lack of clear direction. "There were a lot of different agencies, but it was not clear who was in charge."

The day after the incident, the victims were visited briefly by a group of public health officials from the CDC. The officials told them that the chances that anyone was exposed to anthrax were very remote, but then the officials said they would not know for sure until other laboratory tests were completed in the next few days. Later, when learning more about anthrax, Felice wondered, "In that case, shouldn't we have been taking antibiotics?"

Felice thought that the CDC and other agencies might have gained from inviting the victims to discuss their experience at length. Hearing from the victims could help responders understand the psychological dimension and improve their actions in the future. Four months after the event, when I interviewed Felice, she was still lamenting the lack of such a follow-up. Although the incident was no longer a central concern at the NBC office, "we all watch the mail more cautiously now," she said.

Meanwhile, according to Lieutenant Reggie Lattimer, who led the fire department's response at the NBC site, the experience taught everyone a lot. In the future, he said, "we would not be so quick to have people decontaminated under those circumstances."

Planned Parenthood, Kansas City, Missouri, February 1999

On Monday, February 22, 1999, around 9:30 AM as a snowstorm raged outside, an employee of the Planned Parenthood clinic in midtown Kansas City was opening the mail. She came upon a letter containing brown powder, a skull and crossbones, and a statement that the reader had just been exposed to anthrax. A call to local authorities set in motion a municipal response led by the fire department's HAZMAT team, police, FBI, and medical personnel.[16,17] Before the call was made, a staff member (who asked not to be identified by name) had seen the letter and gone home: "When I saw that dirty-looking piece of paper with a skull and cross bones and the word 'anthrax,' I just left. I did not want to be around." (Personal communication, May 20, 1999.) At home with her three-year-old son, she began to think: "What if I'm infected?" She became increasingly worried and telephoned the clinic. A firefighter told her to take a bath with bleach and water and that someone would call her if there was a problem. About five hours later, she learned from a television broadcast that authorities determined that anthrax apparently was not present. But she remained concerned because "we were not allowed back in the building for two days." (Personal communication, May 20, 1999.)

When firefighters first arrived at the clinic, they quarantined the 20 people who were there and then set up a tent for decontamination outdoors. The detained people—five men and 15 women—were told they would have to undergo a washdown with diluted bleach in the tent. Seven firemen who had entered the building were also ordered to undergo decontamination even though they had been wearing protective gear and masks. The women went through the process first while the 12 men awaited their turns in the building.

One at a time, the victims went outside into the freezing weather. A few men held up tarps to block the view as each victim undressed. Then, completely naked, each victim entered the unheated tent. Once inside, the victim stood in a large basin of water as a woman in a mask and protective gear scrubbed him or her with a bleach and water mixture. Following the scrubbing, the victim was hosed off with cold water. Warm water was not available, according to Chris Bosch, Division Chief of Research/Planning and Emerging Technologies, Kansas City Fire Department. (Personal communication, May 25, 1999.) After decontamination, victims were given disposable blankets to wrap themselves in and then exited the tent. From there, they walked barefoot to an awaiting vehicle. The civilians were brought to a city bus parked nearby and the decontaminated firemen were brought to a HAZMAT truck. Once aboard, they dressed in dry wrappings, sweatsuits, and shoes provided by the Salvation Army.[17] (Personal communication, Greg Ono, Kansas City firefighter, June 16, 1999.)

People were worried and annoyed. "We all were embarrassed to strip," said Ono, who was one of the seven firefighters who went through decontamination, "but some objected more than others." He felt sympathy for one woman in particular, "an older lady who clearly did not want to go out there and undress. She kept coming back into the building—she really felt troubled, but eventually she went." A front-page photograph in *The Kansas City Star* the next day underscored the sense of distress caused by the ordeal. A woman with an anguished expression, wrapped only in a blanket, is shown being escorted to the bus. She is walking barefoot in the icy outdoors with hair soaked from the decontamination wash.[18]

A few days after the event, Christine Vendel, a *Kansas City Star* reporter who covered the incident, received a fax from one of the firemen. He expressed anger about having been forced to undergo the decontamination washdown in the nude by a woman. Vendel said he urged her to write about his being a victim of sexual harassment, but she demurred. (Personal communication, Christine Vendel, May 25, 1999.) None of the three members of the fire department whom I interviewed acknowledged knowing that anyone had sent such a fax.

The event prompted potentially serious health problems for two women who had to be taken to the hospital. After decontamination, one complained of labored breathing and the other became unconscious from an allergic reaction to the bleach solution.[16,17] The psychological impact on many of the victims was profound. Toni Blackwood, chair of the local Planned Parenthood Board, lamented that patients and staff had been "traumatized . . . and terrorized."[16]

Although the Atlanta and Kansas City incidents occurred nearly two years after the B'nai B'rith hoax, actions by local responders were still clearly inappropriate. Indeed, brief reviews of other anthrax threats in 1999 also suggest that inappropriate responses were occurring regularly.

Planned Parenthood Clinic, Boise, Idaho, February 1999

Rebecca Poedy, the financial officer of the Planned Parenthood clinic in Boise, Idaho, opened an anthrax threat letter on Friday afternoon, February 26, 1999. She immediately took it to the clinic director, who called 911. Police detectives were the first to arrive and told her to wash her hands and face. Soon after, with the arrival of medical and fire emergency responders, "there were people all over and it was kind of jumbled," Poedy said. "No one seemed in charge. One of them said to send the staff outside, but others said no, stay in the building." (Personal communication, June 29, 1999.)

Initially, the 24 people in the clinic were kept inside but then were directed outside to the parking lot. After an hour, they were brought inside again and quarantined for another three hours. (Personal communication, Mary McColl, Chief Executive Officer, Planned Parenthood in Boise, Idaho, June 16, 1999.) Meanwhile, the street around the clinic was blocked off. For more than three hours, people in other offices in the area complex were not permitted to leave.[19] Poedy estimates that around 150 people were detained.

Poedy had been kept separate from the others and said she "really began to worry" when firefighters in masks and full gear came for her. They had put up a makeshift shower and wading pool in the middle of the street. A tarp was strung up above the shower, reaching down to knee level. She was instructed to go under the tarp, disrobe, push her clothes out from under the tarp, and shower. After washing with soap and "very cold water," she had to don a white clean suit, gloves, and surgical mask. An ambulance had been summoned and paramedics insisted on placing her in a bodybag before taking her to the hospital. "I objected to the bodybag, but they said I had no other option. They zipped it up to my neck." At the hospital a doctor told her that if she had contracted anthrax, there might be no cure.

Still in mask and gloves, Poedy was made to lie in the bodybag for three hours. She was allowed out only after word was received that initial tests found no evidence of anthrax in the letter. When the shaken Poedy returned to the clinic, Mary McColl, the office's chief executive officer, was distressed about how upset Poedy appeared. McColl had been among the 24 people in the building who were kept isolated. Four months after the incident, McColl said she was still chagrined about Poedy's treatment and her impression that no one seemed in charge. (Personal communication, Mary McColl, June 16, 1999.)

Courthouse, Biloxi, Mississippi, April 1999

On Monday, April 19, 1999, a sheriff's deputy found a note in the parking lot of the county courthouse in Biloxi, Mississippi. It claimed that anthrax had been placed in the building's ventilation system.[20] About 100 people were evacuated and the building remained closed until the next day, according to a reporter who covered the story for *The Sun Herald*. (Personal communication, Blake Kaplan, June 7, 1999.)

The public read about the incident two days later in an article in *The Sun Herald*. Health and law enforcement officials were cited in the article as doubting that anyone had been exposed to anthrax. But an unnerving warning appeared in the article: "As a precaution, however, health officials are warning people who were at the courthouse Monday to be on the lookout for flu-like symptoms such as a cough, runny nose or fever, and to contact their doctor if they have concerns."[20]

The article did not indicate that by the time anthrax symptoms appear, no matter what the treatment, death is likely,[21] nor was there ever a report of how many people might have been in the area, how many thought they might have been exposed, and how many worried if they had a cough and runny nose. According to the reporter who wrote the story, not until one week later was final confirmation received that no harmful biological agents had been present. (Personal communication, Blake Kaplan, June 7, 1999.)

College Office, Syracuse, New York, May 1999

A month later, on Monday, May 17, Robert Duffy was opening the mail in the alumni office at Le Moyne College in Syracuse, New York. When Duffy, the assistant director of the office, unsealed a slightly bulging envelope, a white powder puffed out onto his clothes. "The letter was all folded up so I had to paw around in the envelope and got the stuff all over my hands."[22]

According to Duffy, the letter said: "Anthrax. Congratulations. Death to the Catholics who oppose abortion." (Personal communication, June 8, 1999.) Duffy told his assistant to move away and call security and then he locked himself in his office. After the police arrived, he was told to remain in his office while they evacuated approximately 30 other people who were in the building to an area outside. A Catholic high school across town had just received a similar threat letter and HAZMAT crews were busy over there. Duffy and the people who were detained outside had to remain in place for three hours until the high school was secured. During that time, Duffy was on the telephone answering calls from the FBI, county health officials, and HAZMAT experts. He described the powder to them as "coarse and grainy, like ground-up chalk." Their answer was, "Yes, that's what anthrax looks like."[22]

Panicky, Duffy went on the Internet to learn about anthrax, but the information made him more anxious. "When I read about 90-percent fatality rates, I stopped reading." Three hours later, paramedics arrived in protective gear and masks and told him to undress and wash. Duffy was then dressed in a mask and protective outerwear and brought to an ambulance. (Personal communication, Robert Duffy, June 8, 1999.) His assistant was already in the ambulance and the two were brought to a hospital, where they were scrubbed with soap and water and told to wait. After a few hours, they were informed that tests indicated that anthrax was almost certainly not present.[22]

In recalling the event during an interview a month later, Duffy rued the delayed response. "I was in the office for three hours, waiting," he said. "I think the emergency people should have responded to me sooner." He also said he regretted that authorities did not later contact victims to help with psychological problems brought on by the ordeal.

Other incidents also prompted bizarre, sometimes insensitive responses. After decontamination at an abortion clinic in Arizona, a large woman was given a one-piece white suit to cover herself with. The suit split apart after she put it on, according to a Planned Parenthood worker, but she was told she would have to wear it anyway. (Personal communication, Angie Stefaniak, June 16, 1999.) At a Salt Lake City, Utah, clinic, a victim objected to stripping and being scrubbed with a bleach solution but was told she had no choice. After the bleaching, she was hosed down with cold water as she stood naked, shivering from chill and nervousness. She said the responders tried to be respectful and sensitive, but "I certainly would not go through it again." (Personal communication, Angie Stefaniak, June 16, 1999.)

A woman at a New York City abortion clinic opened a letter on February 22 that read: "Anthrax. Have a nice Death." She called 911. Her impressions after the ensuing six-hour "ordeal," as she put it, were that the responders were serious but disorganized. She posted her concerns on the Internet:

"For example, before I was placed in isolation yesterday [for six hours], I was in the presence of at least 15 police officers and five civilians, all of whom would have been exposed had the threat not proven a hoax. I was faced with ignorance on the part of the police as to how to handle the situation, confusion on the part of the hazardous materials team over what was and was not considered a threat, and in-fighting between agencies that caused dangerous delays."[23] (Statement by Gale Sherman, National Organization of Women (www.now.org/press/02-99/02-23-99.html), posted February 23, 1999.)

Lessons from the Hoaxes

Regrettable as the false bioterrorism alarms have been, they offer immensely valuable lessons. The narratives presented here demonstrate an array of inappropriate emergency responses and the need for consistent, rational behavior by local responders.

1. A uniform response protocol should be made available to local responders. By mid-1999, the CDC and other health associations were issuing sensible advisories. But the information was late in coming and how much was being absorbed by local communities was uncertain. The effectiveness of rehearsals sponsored by the federal government may also be questionable. The emergency responses in two of the communities reviewed above highlight this matter. Federally funded training to respond to a biological or chemical attack had been conducted in Kansas City on January 20–23, 1998, and in Atlanta on March 23–26, 1998.[24] Yet, as shown in this article, their responses to the actual threats the following year were confused and inappropriate.
2. Undressing and showering after a mailed or telephoned bioterrorism threat should not be part of a routine response protocol. Anthrax and other biological agents could be dangerous if inhaled, but if the organisms have already been breathed in, washing skin and clothing would have no effect.
3. Spores that have settled on skin or clothing do not pose an inhalation threat. Any need for surface cleansing can be addressed by washing the hands and face (exposed skin) with soap and water and placing clothing in a plastic bag. Moreover, cutaneous anthrax infection is treatable with antibiotics.
4. Psychological help should be available in the aftermath of an incident. Trained counselors should contact individuals who had particularly stressful experiences such as being forced to undress and undergo scrubbing with bleach solution.
5. Several victims felt that the difficulties of their experiences were compounded by a sense that no one among the emergency responders was in charge. A local response effort needs to be placed under the direction of a single individual whose authority is made obvious to everyone involved.
6. In several cases, integration of responses among various agencies was lacking. Worse, in some instances, open conflict between agency representatives surfaced. The roles of fire, police, HAZMAT, and medical personnel as well as FBI and public health authorities need to be made clear. Local responders should understand where agency responsibilities are distinctive and where they overlap.
7. Some weeks after an incident, victims should be invited to discuss their reactions with appropriate authorities. If victims felt inappropriately treated, their words should be heeded not only as a courtesy but as a means to improve future response approaches.
8. What may have seemed of marginal significance to authorities on the scene was sometimes a matter of profound embarrassment or discomfort to victims. Showering while visible to TV cameras and the public, being doused with extremely hot or extremely cold water, walking barefoot in freezing snow, undergoing decontamination more than once, and being placed in a bodybag after decontamination all left a residue of bitterness and a lack of confidence in the authorities.
9. More rapid laboratory analysis to disconfirm contamination by a bioagent should be made available. In the hoax incidents, definitive findings that anthrax was not present took several days. Delays occurred in part because samples had to be transported to laboratories distant from the incident (to the CDC in Atlanta or the U.S. Army Medical Research Institute of Infectious Diseases at Fort Detrick, Maryland.) Establishing regional laboratories equipped for quick analysis should be a priority.

10. Narratives of incidents involving inappropriate actions such as those recounted in this article should be provided to local responders. The experiences will more likely capture the attention of the authorities for having been real. Moreover, they graphically show what not to do in case of a biothreat.

REFERENCES

1. L.H. Freeh, "The FBI and Weapons of Mass Destruction." http://www.fbi.gov. (13 May 1997.) Accessed January 21, 1999.
2. D.A. Henderson, "The Looming Threat of Bioterrorism," *Science* 283 (1999): 1279–1281.
3. J. Miller and W.J. Broad, "Clinton Describes Terrorism Threat for 21st Century," *The New York Times*, 22 January 1999, sec. A1.
4. S.L. Myers, "U.S. Armed Forces To Be Vaccinated Against Anthrax," *The New York Times*, 16 December 1997, sec. A1.
5. L.A. Cole, "Risks of Publicity about Bioterrorism: Anthrax Hoaxes and Hype," *American Journal of Infection Control* 27, no. 6 (December 1999): 470–473.
6. R.M. Burnham, Federal Bureau of Investigation, Statement for the Record before the U.S. House of Representatives, Subcommittee on Oversight and Investigations. (20 May 1999.)
7. Centers for Disease Control and Prevention, "Bioterrorism Alleging Use of Anthrax and Interim Guidelines for Management—United States, 1998," *Morbidity and Mortality Weekly Report* 48, no. 4 (5 February 1999): 69–74.
8. WMD Operations Unit of the Federal Bureau of Investigation, "Anthrax Advisory." http://www.emergency.com/fbiantrx.htm. (December 1998.) Accessed June 5, 1999.
9. APIC Bioterrorism Task Force, Bioterrorism Readiness Plan: A Template for Healthcare Facilities." Report presented at conference on Bioterrorism, Association for Professionals in Infection Control and Epidemiology, Baltimore, MD, June 24, 1999.
10. M. Keim and A.F. Kaufmann, "Principles for Emergency Response to Bioterrorism," *Annals of Emergency Medicine* 34, no. 2 (August 1999): 177–182.
11. M.L. Wald, "Suspicious Package Prompts 8-Hour Vigil at B'nai B'rith," *The New York Times*, 25 April 1997, sec. A12.
12. Federal Emergency Management Agency, United States Fire Administration, *Fire Department Response to Biological Threat at B'nai B'rith Headquarters*, Washington, DC, April 1997.
13. L.M. Collins and J. Dobner, "An Anthrax Threat at LDL Offices," *Deseret News*, 3 March 1999. http://www.deseretnews.com. Accessed March 5, 1999.
14. V. Coppola, "At War with an Invisible Army," *Atlanta Magazine* (April 1999): 71.
15. E.N. Smith, "Two Packages Purporting to Contain Anthrax Cause Disruptions," *The Atlanta Journal-Constitution*. 4 February 1999. http://www.accessatlanta.com. Accessed February 5, 1999.
16. O. Avila and C. Vendal, "KC Hit by Scare over Anthrax," *The Kansas City Star*, 23 February 1999, sec. A1, A4.
17. Kansas City, Missouri Fire Department, Interdepartmental Communication, After Action Report, 1001 E. 47th Street (Planned Parenthood), March 1, 1999.
18. *The Kansas City Star*, February 23, 1999, sec. A1.
19. L. Wyatt, "Powder Found in Envelope Not Deadly Disease," *The Idaho Statesman*, 27 February 1999, sec. 1A.
20. B. Kaplan, "FBI Investigating Claim," *The Sun Herald*, 21 April 1999. http://www.vh1459.infi.net. Accessed April 21, 1999.
21. A.M. Friedlander, "Anthrax," in *Medical Aspects of Chemical and Biological Warfare*, ed. F.R. Sidell et al. Washington, DC: Borden Institute, Walter Reed Army Medical Center, 1997, 472.
22. S. Weibezahl, "The Letter Hoax a Real Ordeal for Opener," *Herald-Journal* 21 May 1999. http://www.syracuse.com. Accessed May 24, 1999.
23. G. Sherman, National Organization for Women. http://www.now.org/press/02-99/02-23-99.html. (23 February 1999.) Accessed June 5, 1999.
24. Center for Nonproliferation Studies, Monterey Institute of International Studies, "List of Cities with Nunn-Lugar-Domenici Domestic Preparedness Funding with Dates of Completed Training." http://www.cns.miis.edu/research/cbw/120city.htm. (11 December 1998.) Accessed June 7, 1999.

Bioterrorism: Agents of Concern

Theodore J. Cieslak and Edward M. Eitzen, Jr.

The intentional dispersal of biological agents by terrorists is a potential problem that increasingly concerns the intelligence, law enforcement, medical, and public health communities. Terrorists might choose biological agents over conventional and chemical weapons for multiple reasons, although it is difficult to predict, with certainty, which biological agents might prove attractive to terrorists. One can more confidently, however, derive a list of those few agents which, if used, would be of greatest public health consequence. It is these agents which will require the most robust countermeasures. We discuss the derivation of this short list of agents and the specific diseases involved.

Introduction

Biological warfare, according to a definition used during crafting of the 1972 Biological Weapons Convention (BWC), is the "use for hostile purposes of living organisms, whatever their nature, or infective material derived from them, which are intended to cause disease or death in man, animals, or plants."[1(p.18)] While this definition might appear straightforward, little about the topic of biowarfare and bioterrorism is, in reality, without controversy. The very definition follows this pattern and complicates any attempt to develop an "official" list of biological agents of concern.

For example, the former Soviet Union accused the U.S. government of violating the BWC by deploying anti-plant agents such as "Agent Orange" in Southeast Asia. While the U.S. might concede that this constituted anti-plant chemical warfare, it certainly did not fit the U.S. interpretation of the definition of biological warfare. Similarly, the U.S. accused the Soviets of waging biological warfare in those same Southeast Asian jungles by employing trichothecene mycotoxins, a charge the Soviets denied. According to some interpretations, the Soviets considered toxins to fall under the realm of chemical weapons. Recent inquiries into the feasibility of biomodulator

The opinions and assertions contained herein are the private views of the authors and are not to be construed as official or as necessarily reflecting the views of the Department of Defense, the United States Army, or the U.S. Army Medical Research Institute of Infectious Diseases.

Theodore J. Cieslak, MD, *is Staff Physician in the Operational Medicine Division for the United States Army Medical Research Institute of Infectious Diseases in Fort Detrick, Maryland.*

Edward M. Eitzen, Jr., MD, MPH, *is Chief in the Operational Medicine Division for the United States Army Medical Research Institute of Infectious Diseases in Fort Detrick, Maryland.*

(kinins, leukotrienes, substance P, d-sleep-inducing peptide) weaponization, a potential means of warfare in the future according to some analysts, will only serve to heighten this semantic controversy.

Biological warfare is not new and in fact dates at least as far back as 1346.[2] In that year, Tatar invaders laid siege to Kaffa in what is now the Ukrainian Crimea. Defending the city was a group of Genoese merchants. The plague struck the Tatar invaders, who cleverly catapulted bodies of plague victims over the city walls in an attempt to spread plague within the city. The plan appeared to work. The Genoese merchants contracted plague, fled the city, sailed back to Italy, and took the disease with them, firmly establishing the "Black Death" in continental Europe.[2] Given current knowledge, it now seems unlikely that the catapults explain the extension of plague into Kaffa. Bubonic plague is known now to be transmitted by fleas, which rapidly abandon the cooling cadaver. It seems unlikely that corpses catapulted into Kaffa would remain infectious.

American history with biological warfare dates back two centuries to the French and Indian Wars. In 1763, Sir Jeffrey Amherst, commander of British forces in North America, allegedly directed the use of smallpox-laden "gifts" presented to his Indian adversaries.[3] Subsequent outbreaks of smallpox occurred among Native Americans. Like plague, smallpox occupies a prominent position among agents of concern despite its global eradication. Reasons for this are elucidated below.

In the 1930s, the Japanese conducted extensive biological warfare experiments on unwitting civilians and prisoners of war in occupied Manchuria.[4] In response to this and to German research efforts, the U.S. opted in 1943 to establish a biological warfare program of its own at Camp Detrick, Maryland. For the first 10 years, this program was offensive in emphasis, but in 1953, a defensive medical countermeasures program was established. This defensive program remains in place today. A thorough review of the history of biological warfare has recently been published[5] and another is included in this journal issue (see Malloy's article in this issue). In 1969, President Nixon renounced the use of biological weapons by the United States and ordered its offensive program disassembled and its stockpiles destroyed. This destruction occupied the period from 1969–1972 and culminated in the signing of the BWC by the former Soviet Union, the United Kingdom, and the United States. This treaty has since been ratified by more than 140 nations and prohibits the possession, stockpiling, or use of biological weapons.

Developing a Threat List

In order to gain perspective on the nature of a viable bioterrorist weapon, it is useful to consider the agents found in the U.S. arsenal prior to 1969. Ten agents were weaponized in the 1950s and 1960s and are listed in Table 1. These can be grouped into seven antipersonnel agents and three anti-crop agents; the antipersonnel agents are subdivided into lethal agents and incapacitants.[6] A second opinion into the nature of a viable weapon can be sought by consulting Russian sources.[7] A list, in order of priority, of agents considered potential biological weapons by Russian (and presumably Soviet) scientists is provided in the box, "Rating System (Russian) of Bioagent Distribution According to Probability of Use as BW."

Table 1

Destroyed U.S. biological arsenal

Lethal agents	Incapacitating agents	Anti-crop weapons
Bacillus anthracis	Venezuelan equine encephalitis	Wheat-stem rust
Botulinum toxin	Staphylococcal enterotoxin B	Rye-stem rust
Francisella tularensis	*Brucella suis*	Rice-blast spore
	Coxiella burnetii	

Source: Reprinted from U.S. Department of the Army, *U.S. Army Activity in the U.S. Biological Warfare Programs.* Pub. No. B193427L. Washington, DC: U.S. Department of the Army, 1977.

Rating System (Russian) of Bioagent Distribution According to Probability of Use as BW

Smallpox virus
Yersinia pestis
Bacillus anthracis
Botulinum toxin
Venezuelan equine encephalitis virus
Francisella tularensis
Coxiella burnetii
Marburg virus
Influenza virus
Burkholderia mallei
Rickettsia typhi

Source: Reprinted from A.A. Vorobjev et al., "Key Problems of Controlling Especially Dangerous Infections," in *Proceedings of an International Symposium: Severe Infectious Diseases: Epidemiology, Express-Diagnostics and Prevention.* Kirov, Russia: State Scientific Institution, Volgo-Vyatsky Centre of Applied Biotechnology, 1997.

It is useful to consider the biological threat on several levels. From a strategic perspective, biological agents might be used to strike fear into the citizenry of a nation, to diminish the resolve of that citizenry to support war. In this sense, weapons need only be effective enough to instill fear in the population. Perception of a weapon's abilities here might be more important than its actual ability to cause disease. Strategic weapons also might be used against domestic targets important to the conduct of a war abroad such as staging bases, ports of embarkation, command and control assets, and the like. Here, even agents capable of infecting a few key personnel might be strategically effective.

Certain biological agents lend themselves to operational employment. That is, they possess the necessary stability to enable their use over large geographical areas. Fortunately for public health planners, the list of such agents is quite finite. Anthrax, plague, smallpox, tularemia, and perhaps a few other agents might pose viable operational threats. It appears that with some effort, effective countermeasures can be developed against each agent on this short list.

In one sense, the tactical threat is more problematic in that certain viruses and toxins, which lack the stability necessary for effective operational employment, might make adequate tactical weapons. That is, they might be used effectively against smaller, more concentrated targets (such as individual buildings or smaller areas of terrain). Conversely, however, some planners might argue that biological agents are virtually always a poor choice for tactical employment. This stems from the inherent incubation period of biological agents, a characteristic not typically shared by conventional, chemical, and nuclear weapons. This incubation period might vary from hours in the case of staphylococcal enterotoxin B to weeks in the case of brucellosis or Q-fever, but typically is on the order of several days. Commanders tasked with seizing an important terrain objective likely would not want to remain idle while waiting for biological agents to slowly produce their effects. Even if one could envision a tactical use for biological weapons, however, the list of viable candidates remains quite finite, with perhaps fewer than a dozen agents possessing the requisite characteristics.

In considering the terrorist threat, one, in a sense, comes full circle. Here, public perception is again of paramount importance and any attack that might produce headlines can be considered "viable." Moreover, the delay inherent in the incubation period of biological agents likely would be of little concern to the terrorist. The list of available agents thus becomes quite lengthy and the tasks of medical defense planners consequently quite daunting. Agents such as human immunodeficiency virus, rabies, and Ebola, which otherwise might lack characteristics desirable in a weapon, possess the "brand-name" recognition sought by certain terrorists. Similarly, terrorists might select "weapons of opportunity," that is, weapons that might be procured readily by someone in the group. This further lengthens the list of potential agents.

The intentional contamination of restaurant salad bars in The Dalles, Oregon, with Salmonella in 1984 highlights this problem.[8] Although not seriously considered by many military planners, these organisms nonetheless were somewhat effective in the hands of terrorists. Presumably, dozens of other intestinal pathogens and many toxins might be employed similarly. Given these considerations, many in the intelligence and law enforcement communities feel that the magnitude of the terrorist threat, in some ways, surpasses that of the military threat. Moreover, this threat remains nebulous and difficult to monitor adequately. Finally, while response to the military use of such weapons might logically burden defense planners, it is the civilian medical and public health community that would bear the brunt of responding medically to a terrorist release. Consequently, the remainder of this article focuses in greater detail on the nature of this terrorist threat.

Recent U.S. history is filled with examples of the terrorist use of conventional weapons. Beirut, Oklahoma City, Khobar Towers, the World Trade Center, and the American embassies in Nairobi and Dar es Salaam all highlight this threat. Furthermore, the release of Sarin in the Tokyo subway system by members of the Aum Shinrikyo cult is a reminder that terrorists have the ability to procure and deploy chemical weapons as well. Why, then, might terrorists choose a biological weapon? The authors believe that multiple characteristics make biological weapons potentially attractive to terrorists.

First, biological weapons are relatively easy to procure. *Clostridium botulinum*, for example, is ubiquitous in soil and cultured easily by anyone with modest training in microbiology. Ricin is extracted readily from castor beans, which are available throughout the world; recipes for its production are disseminated widely and available on the Internet. Many potential biological weapons, such as *Brucellae* and *Francisella tularensis*, continue to cause endemic disease in many parts of the world. Consequently, clinical laboratories handle cultures of such organisms and constitute a potential source for their acquisition. Culture collections organized for legitimate scientific purposes also may be accessed by those with sinister motives. Four hundred fifty-three such repositories exist in 67 nations; 54 of these sell and ship *Bacillus anthracis*.[9] Devices able to disseminate biological agents are also widely available. Crop-dusting assemblies may be adapted by terrorists for sinister purposes; such devices can, in some cases, generate aerosolized particles of 2–6 μm in diameter, the ideal size for impinging on the human lower respiratory tract.

Second, biological weapons are potentially inexpensive to produce. In 1969, a United Nations panel considered the cost to a belligerent of producing mass (defined as 50%) casualties.[10] To do so over a one-square-kilometer area with conventional weapons would have cost $2,000. Similar destruction wrought by nuclear, chemical, and biological weapons would have cost $800, $600, and $1, respectively.

Third, detection of a biological attack would be problematic. Clouds containing aerosolized biological agents, in contrast to aerosolized chemical weapons, are expected to be odorless, colorless, tasteless, and otherwise invisible. Standoff detection systems are under development but not yet readily available. In fact, initial detection of a bioterrorist attack would not likely involve the finding of explosive devices, missiles, or even crop-dusting equipment, nor would it likely involve environmental detection or the sighting of unusual atmospheric events. Rather, it might involve the widely dispersed presentation to various practitioners, clinics, and emergency departments, of patients with symptoms that are initially nonspecific. This is of grave importance to the clinician because treatment of diseases such as anthrax, plague, botulism, and smallpox is most effective when begun during the incubation period or at least during this early period of nonspecific symptomatology. By the time hallmark findings (mediastinitis in the case of anthrax, hemoptysis in plague victims, neuromuscular symptoms of botulism, the exanthem of smallpox) appear, treatment is of dubious benefit and prognosis is often poor. Moreover, incubation periods ensure that in this age of airline travel, perpetrators can return safely to a foreign land before even nonspecific effects are noticed. Furthermore, contagious diseases such as smallpox and pneumonic plague can continue to propagate, infecting second and third generations of victims prior to discovery and diagnosis.

Finally, biological casualties, more so than conventional or chemical casualties, carry with them the potential to rapidly overwhelm medical capabilities. Botulism, for example, is a survivable disease in the presence of modern medical interventions. Such interventions, however, might include lengthy courses of mechanical ventilation and other intensive care modalities. While these needs are not insurmountable obstacles to the care of an individual patient with endemic foodborne disease, the sudden requirement for hundreds or thousands of intensive care beds in a given city would be extremely difficult to satisfy.

Given these considerations, the authors believe that the possibility of biological terrorism warrants a level of concern and preparedness as great or greater than that devoted to conventional and chemical terrorism. In fact, it is precisely a global lack of preparedness that might magnify the attractiveness of biological weapons in the minds of some terrorists. In certain cases, capitalizing on this lack of preparedness, a terrorist might not need to release or even procure a weapon. The simple threat of release might be enough to influence policy making and government spending. For example, more than 100 anthrax threats have come to the attention of law enforcement agencies during the past two years. As of this writing, every one of these threats was proven to be a hoax.[11] Yet even the most amateur hoax generally leads to a response that may force the expenditure of hundreds of thousands of dollars.

In order to prepare adequately for the possibility of bioterrorism, it is necessary to have some understanding of the specific agents that might be employed by terrorists. A study conducted by the World Health Organization (WHO)[12] demonstrated that anthrax stood alone in its ability to produce mortality. Clearly, if a terrorist group's desire were to cause widespread lethality and assuming the agent could be procured, milled, and delivered optimally, anthrax would seem the weapon of greatest concern. Smallpox, which was not considered in the WHO study, might pose problems of a similar magnitude. In fact, smallpox and pneumonic plague (and to a lesser degree, certain viral hemorrhagic fevers) are noteworthy in that these diseases are contagious—in contrast to most other agents considered here. Terrorists could conceivably leverage the results of an attack by employing these agents as weapons, allowing a very small amount of infectious material to propagate through a population, thus overcoming some of the technical challenges of widespread aerosol delivery (of anthrax, for example).

While certain assumptions and generalizations might be made when attempting to define and combat the terrorist threat, it is clear that the motives and rationale of terrorists cannot always be elucidated. *Shigellae*, *Ascaris suum*, giardia, and schistosomes all have been employed by terrorists, criminals, or other disgruntled persons;[13] it would have been virtually impossible to anticipate and prepare for each of these scenarios. With this in mind, and given the constraint of limited resources, perhaps it is useful to consider not those agents most likely to be used (because this cannot be ascertained) but rather those that, if used, would produce the most devastating consequences and require the most critical medical responses. This is precisely the rationale used recently at the Centers for Disease Control and Prevention (CDC) to develop a list[14] of "critical agents for health preparedness." This list is provided in Table 2. Agents listed as "category A" are those that would have a high overall public health impact and for which intensive public health preparedness and intervention would be necessary. Such preparedness would include a stockpiling of medications and supplies as well as improvements in the current surveillance and response capabilities of local, state, and federal health authorities. Category B agents present a somewhat lesser requirement for preparedness, while category C agents would likely be adequately managed within the framework of the existing public health infrastructure. Only category A agents are considered further here.

The Specific Diseases

Anthrax

Anthrax is caused by infection with *Bacillus anthracis,* a Gram-positive, spore-forming rod. The spore form of this organism is able to survive long periods without nutrients or moisture. It lends itself well to aerosolization, behaves similar to a gas when aerosolized in small particles (drifting readily with air currents), and resists environmental degradation. Moreover, contained within 2–6 micron particles, anthrax spores can be disseminated so as to impinge efficiently on the lower respiratory mucosa, optimizing the chance for infection.

The vast majority of endemic anthrax cases are cutaneous, acquired by close contact with the hides, wool, bone, and other byproducts of infected herbivores (typically cattle, sheep, or goats). Cutaneous anthrax is quite amenable to therapy with many different antibiotics and thus is rarely fatal. While common in parts of Asia and sub-Saharan Africa, it is very rare in the United States, the last case having been reported in 1992. Gastrointestinal anthrax occurs following the consumption of contaminated meat and is likewise quite rare. Inhalational anthrax,

Table 2

Critical agents for health preparedness

Category A	Category B	Category C
Variola virus	*Coxiella burnetii*	All other biological agents my emerge as future threats to public health
Bacillus anthracis	*Brucellae*	
Yersinia pestis	*Burkholderia mallei*	
Botulinum toxin	*Burkholderia pseudomallei*	
Francisella tularensis	Alphaviruses	
Filoviruses and arenaviruses	*Rickettsia prowezekii*	
	Certain toxins (Ricin, SEB)	
	Chlamydia psittaci	
	Food safety threat agents (*Salmonellae*, *E coli* O157:H7)	
	Water safety threat agents (*Vibrio cholera*, etc)	

Source: Reprinted from Centers for Disease Control and Prevention, National Center for Infectious Diseases, *Critical Agents for Health Preparedness, Summary of Selection Process and Recommendations.* Atlanta: CDC, National Center for Infectious Diseases, 1999.

or Woolsorter's disease, was, in the past, an occupational hazard of abattoir and textile workers; immunization has all but eliminated this hazard in western nations. It is this inhalational form of the disease, however, that poses the significant threat of weaponization and employment as an agent of bioterrorism.

Following inhalation of an infectious inoculum (estimated at 8,000–10,000 spores), spores are taken up by pulmonary macrophages. These macrophages carry the spores to regional lymph nodes, most typically in the mediastinum. Within the favorable milieu of the lymph node, *Bacillus anthracis* vegetates and begins to produce edema toxin and lethal toxin. These toxins result in the ultimate necrosis of the lymph node and adjacent tissues, releasing more anthrax organisms, which then gain access to the circulatory system. An overwhelming fatal septicemia rapidly follows. At autopsy, widespread hemorrhage and necrosis, involving multiple organs, is observed.

Anthrax acquired through the inhalational route typically requires an incubation period of one to six days, although incubation periods up to several weeks in length[15] have been reported. Following this, a flu-like illness ensues that is characterized by fever, myalgia, headache, and cough. A brief intervening period of improvement sometimes follows one to two days of these symptoms. Rapid deterioration then ensues; high fever, dyspnea, cyanosis, and shock mark this second phase. Hemorrhagic meningitis occurs in up to 50 percent of cases.[16] Chest radiographs obtained late in the course of illness may reveal a widened mediastinum, and Gram stains of peripheral blood smears may demonstrate the organism at this stage. Prompt treatment is imperative; death occurs in as many as 95 percent of inhalational anthrax cases if such treatment begins more than 48 hours after the onset of symptoms.

A diagnosis of anthrax should be suspected with the finding of sporulating Gram-positive bacilli in skin biopsy material (in the case of cutaneous disease) or in blood smears. Chest radiographs demonstrating a widened mediastinum in the context of fever and constitutional signs—and in the absence of another obvious explanation (such as blunt trauma or post-surgical infection)—also should lead one to consider a diagnosis of anthrax. Confirmation is obtained by blood culture.

Endemic strains of *Bacillus anthracis* are typically sensitive to penicillin G, which remains the drug of choice for endemic anthrax. However, because penicillin-resistant strains of *Bacillus anthracis* can be isolated readily in laboratories, many experts consider ciprofloxacin (400 mg IV q 12 h) the drug of choice for treating victims of intentional anthrax exposure. Doxycycline (100 mg IV q 12 h) is, perhaps, an acceptable alternative, although rare doxycycline-resistant strains of *Bacillus anthracis* have been reported.

Post-exposure prophylaxis against anthrax is accomplished with ciprofloxacin (500 mg PO q 12 h) or doxycycline (100 mg PO q 12 h). Potentially exposed persons should begin receiving antibiotics as soon as possible. In addition, victims should be immunized with chemoprophylaxis administered until a victim has received at least three doses of vaccine, thus, for a minimum of four weeks. Alternatively, 60 days of chemoprophylaxis have been recommended in the absence of immunization.[17] The available vaccine is fully licensed and is given in a six-dose, preexposure regimen at 0, 2, and 4 weeks and at 6, 12, and 18 months. Annual boosters should be administered to persons at continuing risk of exposure. Further recommendations for the management of victims of anthrax terrorism, as well as guidelines for prophylaxis, have recently been published.[11,17]

Anthrax has little potential for person-to-person transmission; standard precautions are adequate for health care workers caring for anthrax victims. Given the one- to six-day incubation period, decontamination of victims presenting days after exposure is probably unnecessary. Re-aerosolization of organisms from skin or clothing likewise poses no significant threat.

Plague

Naturally occurring plague is usually transmitted through the bite of Xenopsylla cheopis, the Oriental rat flea. The causative organism, *Yersinia pestis*, is a bipolar-staining, Gram-negative facultative intracellular bacillus able to survive within the macrophage. This ability aids its dissemination to distant sites following inoculation (or inhalation). It is lymphotrophic and resultant "buboes" (markedly swollen, tender regional lymph nodes) in the distribution of a bite are the hallmark feature of bubonic plague. Virulence factors produced by the organism (such as plasminogen activator) contribute to the spread of bacteria throughout the body. Fever and malaise typically are present among patients with bubonic plague; septicemia often develops as bacteria gain access to the circulation. Eighty percent of bubonic plague victims will have positive blood cultures. Petechiae, purpura, and an overwhelming picture of disseminated intravascular coagulation (DIC) commonly occur. Testimony to the extreme infectivity and lethality of plague can be obtained by considering that the "Black Death" eliminated one-third of the population of Europe during the Middle Ages. Even then, its potential as a weapon was known, as evidenced by its use at Kaffa.

Intentional aerosol dissemination of *Yersinia pestis* would be expected to result in a preponderance of pneumonic plague cases. Pneumonic plague also may arise secondarily after seeding of the lungs of septicemic patients. This disease, along with smallpox, is one of the few bioterrorist threats readily transmissible from person-to-person; coughing patients are often highly contagious. Symptoms of pneumonic plague include fever, chills, malaise, headache, and cough. Chest radiographs may reveal a patchy consolidation and the classic clinical finding is one of blood-streaked sputum. DIC and overwhelming sepsis typically develop as the disease progresses, while meningitis occurs in six percent of cases. Untreated pneumonic plague has a fatality rate approaching 100 percent.

A diagnosis of plague can be suspected by the finding of bipolar "safety-pin" staining bacilli in Gram or Wayson stains of sputum or aspirated lymph node material; confirmation is obtained by culturing Yersinia pestis from blood, sputum, or lymph node aspirate. The organism grows on standard blood or MacConkey's agars, but often is misidentified by automated systems.

Classically, streptomycin (15 mg/kg IM q 12 h) has been considered the drug of choice for treating plague. Gentamicin (1.75 mg/kg IV q 8 h) and doxycycline (100 mg IV q 12 h) are acceptable alternatives. Chloramphenicol should be employed in cases of plague meningitis. In order to be effective, therapy for pneumonic plague must be initiated within 24 hours of the onset of symptoms.

Post-exposure prophylaxis should be provided to asymptomatic victims of a bioterrorist attack as well as to close contacts (including medical personnel) of pneumonic plague patients. Such prophylaxis may be accomplished using tetracycline (500 mg PO qid x 7 d) or doxycycline (or TMP-SMX in the case of tetracycline-intolerant patients). Those in contact with suspected pneumonic plague patients should employ droplet precautions. Such precautions should be continued among patients with confirmed disease until sputum cultures are negative. Standard precautions are appropriate for managing bubonic plague victims. Because of the plague's incubation period, decontamination would rarely be required in a clinical setting. A plague vaccine exists but currently is out of production. The vaccine was developed to prevent bubonic plague in endemic regions and, based on animal data, is unlikely to protect against pneumonic plague.

Smallpox

The eradication of smallpox surely ranks as one of the greatest success stories in the history of public health, with the last endemic case occurring in Somalia in 1977. Since then, research stockpiles of variola virus have been maintained at two maximum-security WHO-approved sites: the CDC in Atlanta and the State Research Center of Virology and Biotechnology, a Russian institute near Novosibirsk. Although this would seem to make terrorist employment of this virus impossible, several factors give cause for concern. First is the fear that other stockpiles already exist in the hands of belligerent nations. Second, the entire viral genomic sequence is known and published, making it possible that technology soon might permit reconstruction of the virus. Finally, although the virulence factors of variola virus are poorly understood, it may be possible for someone to manipulate related orthopoxviruses such as Monkeypox, thereby enhancing their virulence in humans.[18]

Multiple factors might make smallpox an attractive weapon to potential terrorists. Immunity following vaccination may last only three to five years. Moreover, vaccine is no longer in production and current stockpiles are dwindling and/or losing potency. Susceptibility to smallpox is universal, even among those vaccinated in the past. There is no effective therapy for smallpox and modern health care providers are unfamiliar with the disease. Finally, the potential for rapid spread potentially permits a terrorist to cause widespread disease and panic with a minimum of infectious material.

The incubation period of smallpox is 7–17 days. This would permit wide dispersal of exposed persons before signs and symptoms appear. During the incubation period, virus replicates in the upper respiratory tract, ultimately giving rise to a primary viremia. Amplification of virus occurs following seeding of the liver and spleen and a secondary viremia then develops. The skin is seeded during this secondary viremia and the classic exanthem of smallpox appears.

During the phase of secondary viremia, clinical illness begins abruptly and is characterized by fever, rigors, vomiting, headache, backache, and extreme malaise. The classical exanthem begins two to four days later. Macules are seen initially on the face and extremities; these macules progress in synchronous fashion to papules, then to pustules, and finally to scabs. As these scabs separate, survivors can be left with disfiguring, de-pigmented scars. The synchronous nature of the rash and its centrifugal distribution distinguish smallpox from chickenpox, which has a centripetal distribution. Death occurs in 30 percent of variola major (the predominant form of smallpox in the past) patients and typically results from concomitant visceral organ involvement. Eye involvement leads to blindness in a small number of victims. In addition to classical variola major, uncommon variants with lesser (variola minor) or greater (hemorrhagic, flat-type smallpox) mortality were described during the smallpox era.

A single case of smallpox occurring anywhere in the world today would represent the gravest of public health emergencies, and suspicion should prompt immediate consultation with health authorities. Strict quarantine (airborne and contact precautions in current terminology) should be instituted immediately for victims (until all scabs separate) as well their contacts (for 17 days from last exposure). Multiple victims ideally would be managed as a cohort at dedicated sites removed from conventional hospital facilities.

Based on past experience, vaccination of smallpox-exposed persons within the first several days after exposure would be efficacious in preventing disease. Vaccinia (an orthopoxvirus related to variola and useful in inducing immunity to other orthopoxviruses) vaccine may be obtained through the CDC. Although successful at eradicating smallpox, vaccinia administration is fraught with complications. In order to manage these complications, vaccinia immune globulin (VIG) must be stockpiled when undertaking a vaccination campaign. VIG (0.6 mg/kg IM) may be given to vaccine recipients who experience severe complications or to significantly immunocompromised individuals exposed to smallpox, in whom vaccination would be unsafe. In addition to the limited availability of vaccine, extremely limited supplies of VIG hamper any response plan. Additional guidelines for the medical and public health management of an intentional smallpox release have recently been published.[19]

Botulism

Botulism occurs following exposure to one of seven related botulinum neurotoxins (A–G) produced by certain strains of *Clostridium botulinum*, a strictly anaerobic spore-forming, Gram-positive bacillus commonly found in soil. These neurotoxins are the most toxic substances known, with an LD_{50} (for type A toxin) of 0.001 μg/kg. They function at the presynaptic nerve terminal, preventing the release of acetylcholine and thereby leading to a generalized flaccid paralysis and autonomic dysfunction. Only types A, B, and E toxin appear to be significant causes of naturally occurring human botulism, although other serotypes have the potential to cause human disease. For this reason, a licensed antitoxin having activity only against these three serotypes is produced.

After exposure to botulinum toxin, a latent period ranging from 24 hours to several days is required before clinical manifestations develop. Signs and symptoms initially involve cranial nerve dysfunction, manifested as bulbar palsies, ptosis, photophobia, and blurred vision owing to difficulty in accommodation. Symptoms then progress to include dysarthria, dysphonia, and dysphagia. Finally, a descending symmetric paralysis develops and death may result from respiratory muscle failure.

A solitary case of botulism must be differentiated from other uncommon neurological disorders such as myasthenia gravis and Guillain-Barré syndrome. The presence of multiple casualties with similar symptoms clustered in time and space should make elucidation of a botulism outbreak relatively easy. Supportive care, with meticulous attention to ventilatory support, remains the mainstay of botulism management. Patients may require such support for several months, making the management of a large-scale botulism outbreak especially problematic in terms of medical resources.

A licensed trivalent (types A, B, E) botulinum antitoxin is available through the CDC. Although administration of antitoxin is unlikely to reverse disease, it may prevent progression when administered to exposed persons. Botulinum antitoxin is prepared from horse serum; a test dose thus should be administered before therapy. Patients reacting to a test dose require desensitization prior to treatment. An investigational heptavalent despeciated (F_{ab2}) antitoxin, also produced in horses, is available through the U.S. Army Medical Research Institute of Infectious Diseases on a compassionate use protocol.[20] Administration of a test dose also is required with this product.

Tularemia

Tularemia is a highly infectious disease caused by the Gram-negative *coccobacillus*, *Francisella tularensis*. The very low inoculum required for infection (estimated to be 10 or fewer organisms) as well as its survivability in the environment contribute to its inclusion on the list of agents of concern. Several clinical forms of endemic tularemia are known but inhalational exposure in a terrorist attack would likely lead to pneumonia or to the typhoidal form of the disease, manifested as a variety of nonspecific symptoms including fever, malaise, and abdominal pain. Streptomycin or gentamicin, in doses similar to those recommended for plague, is recommended as therapy. Post-exposure prophylaxis consists of doxycycline, tetracycline, or ciprofloxacin administered for two weeks.

Viral hemorrhagic fevers

The viral hemorrhagic fevers are a heterogeneous group of diseases caused by lipid-enveloped RNA viruses belonging to one of four taxonomic families: (1) the Arenaviridae, (2) Filoviridae, (3) Flaviviridae, and (4) Bunyaviridae. While the diseases produced by these agents differ considerably in their clinical manifestations, severity, and modes of transmission, they share a propensity to cause a bleeding diathesis. The severity of hemorrhagic manifestations also varies considerably among the various viruses but all are potentially infectious by the aerosol route and most are stable as respirable aerosols. These factors make them agents of concern from a terrorism perspective. The potential for human-to-human transmission makes the filoviruses (such as Ebola and Marburg viruses) and arenaviruses (such as Lassa Fever Virus) particularly concerning. Therapy of the various viral hemorrhagic fevers is principally supportive in nature, although intravenous ribavirin appears somewhat efficacious in treating arenaviral disease. A licensed vaccine is available only for one agent, namely, Yellow Fever Virus, a flavivirus.

■ ■ ■

The potential use of biological agents as vehicles for terrorism remains a high-priority concern of military, government, and civilian planners as well as public health authorities. These authorities, as well as clinicians and emergency personnel, at a minimum need to develop a heightened sense of awareness and clinical acumen regarding the management of a biological attack. While it is virtually impossible to predict which agents a terrorist might employ, it is possible to derive a list of those agents that, *if employed*, would present the greatest potential for catastrophe. Clinicians and public health authorities must have a working knowledge of the diagnosis, pathogenesis, and treatment of the diseases caused by these agents.

REFERENCES

1. N.A. Sims, *The Diplomacy of Biological Disarmament*. New York: St. Martin's Press, 1988.
2. V.J. Derbes, "De Mussis and the Great Plague of 1348: A Forgotten Episode of Bacteriological War," *JAMA* 196 (1966): 59–62.
3. F. Parkman, *The Conspiracy of Pontiac and the Indian War after the Conquest of Canada*. Boston: Little, Brown, and Co., 1901.
4. S. Harris. "Japanese Biological Warfare Research on Humans: A Case Study of Microbiology and Ethics," *Annals of the New York Academy of Sciences* 666 (1992): 21–52.
5. G.W. Christopher, et al., "Biological Warfare: A Historical Perspective," *JAMA* 278 (1997): 412–417.
6. U.S. Department of the Army, *U.S. Army Activity in the U.S. Biological Warfare Programs*. Pub. No. DTIC B193427L. Washington, DC: U.S. Department of the Army, 1977.
7. A.A. Vorobjev, et al., "Key Problems of Controlling Especially Dangerous Infections," in *Proceedings of an International Symposium: Severe Infectious Diseases: Epidemiology, Express-Diagnostics and Prevention*. Kirov, Russia: State Scientific Institution, 1997.
8. T.J. Torok, et al., "A Large Community Outbreak of Salmonellosis Caused by Intentional Contamination of Restaurant Salad Bars," *JAMA* 278 (1997): 389–395.
9. R.M. Atlas, "Biological Weapons Pose Challenge for Microbiology Community," *ASM News* 64 (1998): 383–389.
10. Departments of the Army, Navy, and Air Force, *NATO Handbook on the Medical Aspects of NBC Defensive Operations (AMedP-6(B)*. Washington, DC: Departments of the Army, Navy, and Air Force, 1996.
11. Centers for Disease Control and Prevention, "Bioterrorism Alleging Use of Anthrax and Interim Guidelines for Management—United States, 1998," *Morbidity and Mortality Weekly Report* 48 (1999): 69–74.
12. World Health Organization, *Health Aspects of Chemical and Biological Weapons*. Geneva, Switzerland: World Health Organization, 1970.
13. W.S. Carus, *Bioterrorism and Biocrimes: The Illicit Use of Biological Agents in the 20th Century*. Washington, DC: National Defense University, 1999.
14. Centers for Disease Control and Prevention, National Center for Infectious Diseases, *Critical Agents for Health Preparedness, Summary of Selection Process and Recommendations*. Atlanta: Centers for Disease Control and Prevention, National Center for Infectious Diseases, 1999.
15. M. Meselson, et al., "The Sverdlovsk Anthrax Outbreak of 1979," *Science* 266 (1994): 1202–1208.
16. F.A. Abramova, et al., "Pathology of Inhalational Anthrax in 42 Cases from the Sverdlovsk Outbreak of 1979," *Proceedings of the National Academy of Sciences of the USA*, 90 (1993): 2291–2294.
17. T.V. Inglesby, et al., "Anthrax as a Biological Weapon," *JAMA* 281 (1999): 1735–1745.
18. J.G. Bremen and D.A. Henderson, "Poxvirus Dilemmas—Monkeypox, Smallpox, and Biological Terrorism," *New England Journal of Medicine* 339 (1998): 556–559.
19. D.A. Henderson, et al., "Smallpox as a Biological Weapon," *JAMA* 281 (1999): 2127–2137.
20. R.G. Hibbs, et al., "Experience with the Use of an Investigational $F(ab')_2$ Heptavalent Botulism Immune Globulin of Equine Origin During an Outbreak of Type E Botulism in Egypt," *Clinical Infectious Disease* 23 (1996): 337–340.

A History of Biological and Chemical Warfare and Terrorism

Curtis D. Malloy

This article provides a brief history of biological warfare and terrorism. It contends that examining disease in history provides public health specialists with the knowledge necessary to improve our surveillance system for potential acts of bioterrorism.

VIEWED THROUGH the lens of history, natural disease transmission and anthropogenic epidemics can be difficult to distinguish. Furthermore, assessing the differences between acts of warfare and those with terrorist intent can present an even greater challenge. As civilian populations were often geographically intermixed with combatants, an event intended to inflict disease on a military objective often resulted in collateral casualties among civilians. Military objectives thus were obtained through acts of both warfare and terrorism. Terror also played an important role in these man-made epidemics, as those fleeing disease often inadvertently contributed to its propagation.

Allegations of terrorism—whether it employs a biological agent, chemical agent, entomological agent, or a combination of the three—are inherently difficult to confirm. Authentication of historical events is more often impossible due to an absence of epidemiological and microbiological evidence and an unwillingness by the perpetrators to diminish their cause through admitting the use of such tactics. Medical historians therefore have relied on bystander observations, correspondence, and art forms (tapestries, pottery images, and paintings) to substantiate allegations.

Perhaps the first reference to epidemics, intoxications, and environmental manipulation used with coercive intent could be traced to the Ten Plagues of Egypt in the Hebrew Bible's book of *Exodus*.[1,2] In this compelling narrative, a story unfolds that describes God in two apparently conflicting roles—that of

The author would like to express his gratitude to Amy Knight, MPH, and Diane Monroe for their review of this manuscript.

Curtis D. Malloy, MPH, *is a consultant living in Seattle, Washington.*

"hardening the Pharaoh's heart" so the Pharaoh would be disinclined to accept the entreaties of Moses to "Let my people go" and that of incurring devastating retribution to the Egyptians for keeping the Israelites enslaved.[3,4] After a series of environmental catastrophes, epidemics, epizootics, zoonotics, and intoxications,[5] the Pharaoh eventually was forced to submit to Moses' demands.

The Hebrew Bible contains two additional references to what could be construed as anti-crop attacks. *Judges* 9:45 tells of the use of salt to poison the soil:

> ... Abimelech fought against the city all that day; and he took the city, and slew the people that [were] therein, and beat down the city, and sowed it with salt.[1(p.253)]

Just six chapters later (*Judges* 15:9), the narrative indicates:

> ... Samson went and caught three hundred foxes, and took firebrands, and turned tail to tail, and put a firebrand in the midst between two tails. And when he had set the brands on fire, he let [them] go into the standing corn of the Philistines, and burnt up both the shocks, and also the standing corn, with the vineyards [and] olives.[1(p.258–259)]

While a chemical is used in the former incident to limit the capacity of land to bear fruit, the latter reference appears to be the earliest extant reference to the use of biological vectors (foxes) with intent to damage crops.

In addition to events in the Hebrew Bible, the strategic use of biological and chemical agents has permeated the history of warfare. The use of animal and human cadavers to contaminate potable water supplies has been documented in Persian, Greek, and Roman literature beginning in 300 BC.[6] (Such attempts to contaminate water supplies must have held strategic advantages as similar acts were documented among Confederate soldiers during the United States' Civil War.[7])

During the Battle of Eurymedon, Hannibal was purported to have used catapults to launch earthen pots filled with poisonous snakes into King Eumenese II of Pergamon's flagship—a prescient example of airborne biological weaponry.[8] In the 14th century, as the Tatar forces besieged the city of Kaffa (now Feodossia, Ukraine), the cadavers of plague victims were catapulted over the city's walls. Whether the intent was to promote the spread of bubonic plague or to terrorize the inhabitants of the walled city, the second pandemic of plague commenced shortly thereafter. The efficacy of human projectiles as fomites for plague has been questioned as fleas are known to abandon dead bodies rapidly.[8] The epidemic within and without the besieged city was more probably the product of co-exposure to rats and their infected fleas. The use of such tactics appears to have been commonplace given the plentitude of classical tapestries illustrating the practice of launching human remains over cities under siege.[7]

In 1650, a Polish infantryman suggested the use of airborne biological warfare in the form of modified bomblets, constructed by engineering "hollow spheres filled with the slobber of rabid dogs and other substances that can poison the atmosphere and cause epidemics."[9(p.512–513)] This event has been cited as representing early concepts in the aerosolization of infectious agents and, implicitly, the dissemination of chemical warfare agents.[9]

During the French and Indian War in 1763, the commander of the British forces in North America, Sir Jeffrey Amherst, advocated the use of one of today's most feared biological agents. In a communication with his ranking field commander, Colonel Henry Bouquet, Amherst sent a note with the following query:

> Could it not be Contrived to Send the Small Pox among those Disaffected Tribes of Indians? We must, on this occasion, use Every Stratagem in our power to Reduce them.[7(p.12)]

Bouquet responded with the handwritten statement:

> I will try to inoculate the — with Some Blankets that may fall in their Hands, and take care not to get the disease myself.[7(p.12)]

It has been interpreted that Bouquet not using the word "Indian" represented an implicit acknowledgment of the disapproval such an undertaking would have provoked among outside observers.[7] Furthermore, the comment was handwritten at the bottom of the correspondence, apparently to ensure the office redactor would not see the controversial exchange.[7] Amherst replied with implicit approval of the plan, stating:

> You will Do well to try to Inoculate the Indians, by means of Blankets, as well as Try Every other Methode, that can Serve to Extirpate this Execrable Race.[7(p.12)]

In the American Revolutionary War, natural disease transmission and vaccination played a crucial role as British troops underwent variolation against smallpox. American colonists did not receive similar prevention methods until General Washington ordered a wholesale vaccination campaign later in the war.[10]

World War I saw the effective, yet tragic addition of chemicals to conventional warfare. Chemical agents—first chlorine and later phosgene and mustard gas—killed or injured more than one million soldiers and civilians.[11] Attempting to limit the transport of pack animals and food to Europe, German saboteurs allegedly infected mules, cattle, and horses with both anthrax and glanders in both Argentina and the United States.[6]

During the First World War, the perceived dangers presented by biological and chemical warfare had a profound effect on the social conscience—so much so in fact that rumors circulated that the "Spanish" Influenza of 1918 was the product of German biological warfare. Some theories posited that the causal pathogen was placed into Bayer aspirins (the product of a German pharmaceutical company) and disseminated through intentional product contamination.[12]

Following World War I, the 1925 Geneva Protocol for the Prohibition of the Use in War of Asphyxiating, Poisonous or Other Gases, and of Bacteriological Methods of Warfare was initiated. Many nations reserved the right to respond in kind to the use of biological warfare agents and the treaty did not address the issue of research and development of agents or the production and stockpiling of pathogens and delivery systems.[7] The United States Senate did not ratify the Geneva Protocol until 1975.[6]

Prior to World War II, Japan began conducting experiments in Manchuria with an array of diseases including plague, anthrax, typhus, and cholera.[13] Toxins associated with poisonous snakes and blowfish also were examined for their strategic value.[13] Under the supervision of Generals Shiro Ishii and Kitano Misaji, the Japanese military built several biological warfare facilities that eventually employed more than 3,000 scientists and technicians.

Japanese research rapidly progressed from basic science to the use of prisoners as human subjects. At least 10,000 victims, mostly Chinese, were exposed to organisms that cause plague, smallpox, anthrax, yellow fever, typhus, tularemia, hepatitis, gas gangrene, cholera, tetanus, glanders, dysentery, scarlet fever, tick encephalitis, diphtheria, pneumonia, typhoid fever tuberculosis, venereal diseases, Salmonellosis, and others.[13] The human subjects were either killed by the pathogens or by their captors; none were allowed to survive. The Japanese tested their research during several attacks on civilian and military populations: nearby cities were exposed systematically to plague, cholera, and typhus. In Nanking, China, Ishii had chocolates infused with anthrax spores distributed to children to determine if this method of spread was suitable for other uses.[13] The Japanese engaged in entomological warfare as well, scattering plague-infected fleas in areas that shortly thereafter saw localized, but deadly, epidemics. In 1939, "suicide squads" were sent into Outer Mongolia and Russia to infect sheep and cattle with anthrax and other diseases.[13] Anti-crop agents (pesticides and herbicides) also were evaluated for their efficacy.[13]

During this same period, historical references are silent regarding the use of biological and chemical weapons in the war in Europe. However, one should consider the use of Zyclon B to kill six million Jews and other victims as an act of counter-civilian terrorism. There was great concern among Allied powers that the Germans would use chemical or biological agents in the field. In actuality, Adolph Hitler had suspended such research by the year 1939.[8] In the latter portion of the war, this suspension was superceded as experimentation was undertaken by Nazi physicians on those held in concentration camps; victims were exposed to *Rickettsia prowazekii, Rickettsia mooseri*, Hepatitis A virus, and *Plasmodia spp* and experimental vaccines and drugs were administered.[6] It is unclear whether the motivation of this research was to engage in biological weapons research or merely to advance basic science—independent of the motivation, the actions were condemned rightfully during the Nuremberg trials.

In response to fears that soldiers would be susceptible to a biological weapon employing yellow fever, Allied soldiers were inoculated with an unlicensed vaccine. Any soldier who refused vaccination was subject to court-martial. Due to a contamination in the stocks of vaccines, which contained human sera, at least 51,000 military personnel were hospitalized with Hepatitis B infection in 1942 and estimates of those infected soared to 330,000 individuals.[14] With an eye toward this unfortunate debacle, a debate currently is underway on the wisdom and efficacy of requiring vaccination to prevent inhalational anthrax among members of the United States armed forces.[15,16]

The United States commenced its own research into biological and chemical agents in 1941 through its Chemical Warfare Service. George W. Merck, president of the pharmaceutical company Merck & Co., Inc., was named the civilian head of the agency. The program changed its name to the War Research Service in 1942 and examined anthrax and botulism for their effectiveness as agents for biological warfare; anti-crop agents also were studied. The total cost of the United States' biological warfare program was approximately $60 million compared with the $2 billion budget for the Manhattan Project.[17]

Evidence exists that President Franklin D. Roosevelt, Admiral William Leahy, and other advisors discussed utilizing anti-crop agents against the Japanese rice harvest in 1944; the idea was scrapped because some advisors felt the effect of the destruction of the 1945 rice crop would not yield military results until well into 1946. After the end of the war, President Truman indicated in a letter to an advisor that if the war in the Pacific had continued past mid-August 1945, he would have considered employing chemical and biological weaponry.[17]

In World War II Poland, an altruistic biological "war" was waged by two Polish physicians, Lazowski and Matulewicz.[18] These largely unrecognized physicians purposefully infected patients with the non-pathogenic soil bacterium *Proteus*, which elicited an immune response to *Rickettsia prowazeki*. Upon seeing false-positive laboratory response, the Gestapo, fearing an outbreak of typhus in Germany where one had not occurred in more than a quarter of a century, abandoned attempts to deport individuals from 12 surrounding villages.[19] (Personal communication, E.S. Lazowski, Assistant Professor Emeritus, University of Illinois, December 17, 1999.)

During the conflict in Korea, initially North Korea and later China charged that the United States-led United Nations forces were deploying chemical, biological, and entomological agents.[20,21] Among the vectors that the communists claimed were dispersed were ants, bees, black beetles, butterflies, caterpillars, crickets, field crickets, fleas, flies, lice, locusts, mites, mosquitoes, sandflies, spiders, and springtails.[20] The diseases supposedly spread were anthrax, cholera, dysentery, encephalitis, paratyphoid, plague, rickettsia, smallpox, typhoid, and typhus.[20] The evidence provided by the communist health officials included witnesses, laboratory tests, autopsies, and data indicating seasonal variations in insect density.[20] Both the United States and the United Nations denied the allegations.

Such allegations continued during the Vietnam War, with the United States claiming that North Vietnam was using tricothecene mycotoxins in a campaign in Laos.[22] Similar to the allegations made during the Korean conflict, these claims of "yellow rain" never were substantiated. The Vietnam War also saw the use of more primitive, but at times still effective, uses of biological weaponry: in the early 1960s—the Viet Cong utilized booby-trapped "pungi" sticks smeared with excrement.[6]

The Cold War—with the main participants being the United States and the former Soviet Union—accompanied a monumental increase in the body of knowledge related to biological warfare and terrorism. The United States government's sense of vulnerability led it to well-documented research of simulants on its own constituency.[2,23–25]

The first of a series of questionable domestic experiments using non-consenting human subjects in chemical and biological simulant studies began in 1949 when the United States military "attacked" its own headquarters: *Serratia marcescens* was systematically sprayed into the Pentagon's intake vents. The success of the mission—measured by the extent to which the simulant spread into many areas of the facility—convinced the military of the magnitude of the threat posed by biochemical warfare and terrorism and reinforced the decision to continue with a simulant program.[2]

Continuing its research on pathogens and the dispersive capacity of biological and chemical agents, Camp Detrick's Special Operations division used *Serratia marcescens* and *Bacillus globigii* as simulants. Extensive tests, now well documented with data gathered using the Freedom of Information Act, were undertaken on unknowing civilian populations in Virginia, San Francisco, New York, and other locations from 1949 to 1960.[2] A number of deaths due to *Serratia marcescens* at Stanford University demonstrated a temporality consistent with tests using this simulant in nearby San Francisco. However, several factors minimized the likelihood of a causal relation between the military's use of Serratia marcescens and clusters of subsequent cases—including the fact that all the Stanford patients had undergone urinary tract catheterization and that the strains isolated did not match the 8UK strain used by the U.S. Army.[6] Despite a panel recommending that a less pathogenic simulant be utilized, studies with *Serratia marcescens* continued until 1968.[6]

The U.S. Army also used *Bacillus globigii* as a simulant, in some cases dispersing the agent in the New York City subway system. This research on the vulnerability of subway systems is not historically unique: similar reports exist of *Serratia marcescens* used as a simulant by Nazis in 1932 in the Paris subway system[25] as well as by the Soviets in the Moscow subway system during the 1980s.[26]

A series of investigations conducted by the Army Chemical Corps termed Operation LAC (Large Area Coverage) demonstrated the nation's level of vulnerability to the airborne dispersal of biological and chemical agents. In 1958, the Air Force loaned the Army Chemical Corps a C-119 "flying boxcar," which was used to release zinc cadmium sulfide by the ton in the atmosphere above the Midwestern United States. The research was designed to determine the dispersion of agents and their potential geographic range as the fluorescent particles were traced by ground stations throughout the United States. Particles were detected up to 1,200 miles from the drop point.[2]

By the late 1950s, the U.S. military extended its investigations to the use of entomological agents in warfare. Operation "Big Itch" assessed the problems associated with cultivating and dropping munitions loaded with fleas; the tests were considered a success. Operation "Big Buzz" assessed the limitations of using the Aedes aegypti mosquito as a vector of yellow fever. In this experiment, approximately one million uninfected females were produced and released in Georgia. Further experimentation under the code name Project Whitecoat used human volunteers, most of whom were members of the 7th Day Adventists; these participants were largely conscientious objectors willing to participate in non-combatant Army research.[25]

In 1969, President Nixon announced the unilateral decision to discontinue offensive biological research and destroy the United States' arsenal, stating:

> Mankind already carries in its own hands too many of the seeds of its own destruction. By the examples we set today, we hope to contribute to an atmosphere of peace and understanding between nations and among men.[27(p.93)]

The order also mandated that all existing stocks of biological warfare agents be destroyed. Many analysts have disputed the capacity to differentiate between offensive and defensive research in biological warfare; others have made the claim that President Nixon's decision was based more on politics and an ambiguous return on the United States' investment in biological research.[2] Critics also point to the fact that the U.S. supply of agents and toxins was difficult to contain and posed a risk to military personnel and nearby civilians—for example, the year before President Nixon's declaration, an accident with nerve agents killed 6,000 sheep in Utah.[2] Nevertheless, in 1972, the multinational Biological Weapons Convention was signed banning the production of biological pathogens and their toxins.

The former Soviet Union's research into weapons of biological warfare allegedly began in 1928, with typhus representing the first agent examined for battlefield efficacy. Unconfirmed reports indicate that the former Soviet Union's biological warfare program was behind an outbreak of Q fever in the Crimea in 1943.[26] During the next 60 years, the program evolved into the research arm of the military known as "Biopreparat;" the personnel employed may have included up to 50,000 microbiologists, physicians, engineers, and other nontechnical personnel.[28] Following the end of World War II, the former Soviet Union obtained data from Japanese biological research facilities in Manchuria, which assisted in the military's growing commitment to biological weaponry.[26] The Soviet system examined the suitability of a broad array of chemical, biological, and anti-crop pathogens.

In 1980, reports began to emerge from the former Soviet Union that a civilian community in the Sverdlovsk region had experienced an outbreak of anthrax. Initial reports released by Soviet medical, veterinary, and legal journals claimed an outbreak occurred in March and April 1979, which was largely gastrointestinal in manifestation. The official report claimed that contaminated meat from infected disease was to blame and several persons were arrested and charged with selling tainted meat on the black market. Independent international researchers determined that at least 77 cases occurred, of which 66 victims died. A geographic analysis of the event, coupled with atmospheric data for the period in question, resulted in the hypothesis that nearby Military Compound 19 may have released an airborne plume of anthrax spores.[29] In 1992, Russian President Boris Yeltsin, who at the time of the outbreak was the chief Communist Party official in Sverdlovsk, admitted the epidemic was indeed the result of an unintentional release of anthrax from the research facility. The event in Sverdlovsk is considered the largest documented epidemic of inhalational anthrax.[6]

Iraq initiated its biological warfare program in 1974 and expanded its research dramatically in 1985. The Iraqi program investigated a number of pathogens, including five bacterial agents, one fungus, five viruses, and four toxins. Research was conducted to weaponize and deliver biological and chemical payloads, and by the commencement of the Persian Gulf War in 1992, Iraq had deployed approximately 200 bombs and 25 ballistic missiles containing biological agents.[30,31] Iraq also possessed chemical and nerve warfare agents, which it employed in 1982–1983 during the Iran/Iraq War.[2]

Actions that are perpetrated by an individual for immediate gain (financial, coercive, or merely personal vengeance) often are construed as acts of terrorism. In 1982, a series of deaths in Chicago suburbs alerted public health officials to a threat due to the purposeful chemical contamination of packaged goods. Seven persons died and several more were hospitalized with cyanide poisoning after ingesting Extra-Strength Tylenol capsules.[32] While intentional food poisoning is not a new phenomenon—Philip of Macedon is said to have arranged the poisoning of Aratus the elder in the third century, BC—the public's sense of vulnerability sparked a massive engineering move toward tamper-resistant packaging.[33,34]

In the fall of 1984, a large community outbreak of foodborne disease occurred in The Dalles, Oregon. Epidemiological investigations of the incident indicated *Salmonella Typhimurium* as the causal agent.[35] A criminal investigation linked the *Salmonella Typhimurium* to laboratories owned by followers of Bhagwan Shree Rajneesh. In March 1986, two members of the Rajneesh commune were indicted for conspiring to tamper with consumer products by pouring cultures of *Salmonella Typhimurium* onto items at restaurant salad bars and into coffee creamer containers. Prosecutors accused the followers of attempting to incapacitate voters in an upcoming election: the members pled guilty and were sentenced to four and one half years in prison.

During March 1995, the Tokyo subway system came under chemical attack by the cult Aum Shinrikyo using Sarin gas. Investigations of the cult's activities revealed that other attacks had been attempted using pathogens (anthrax spores, cholera, and Q fever), biological toxins (botulinum), and chemical agents. The group previously had traveled to the former country of Zaire with the intention of obtaining isolates of the Ebola virus.[36]

In October 1996, muffins and doughnuts anonymously left for laboratory personnel in a staff room of a Texas hospital sickened 12 laboratory workers. *Shigella dysenteriae* type 2 was cultured from the stool of nine patients, and the isolates were identical to that recovered from an uneaten muffin and linked to the laboratory's stock strain.[37] A laboratory technician admitted to intentionally exposing her coworkers and then admitted to similarly infecting her boyfriend and switching a laboratory sample of his stool to avoid detection.[38]

A comparable event occurred in 1998 when 67 people became ill after eating curry at a summer festival in Wakayama, Japan. Following the death of four persons, doctors initially diagnosed food poisoning, then cyanide poisoning, and then arsenic poisoning.[39] Similar events have occurred in Japan using cyanide, sodium azide, and cresol in Tokyo, Nagano, Osaka, Kyoto, and Okazaki.[40,41] While the mass-poisoning in Wakayama instilled terror in the population, the intent was allegedly to perpetrate insurance fraud.[42] The motivations behind the latter events have not been determined.

■ ■ ■

Examining disease in history provides public health specialists important insight into the origins of diseases, the manner in which they spread, and the probable causes of numerous epidemics of antiquity.[43–45] The history of biological warfare and terrorism is not merely a retrospective view of past incidences but also an opportunity to examine historic events with an eye toward predicting the future. Our knowledge of the past informs our surveillance system for potential acts of contemporary biological warfare and terrorism.

REFERENCES

1. *The Holy Bible*, King James Version. New York: Harper Paperbacks, 1995.
2. L.A. Cole, *The Eleventh Plague: The Politics of Biological and Chemical Warfare*. New York: WH Freeman and Company, 1997.
3. G. Hort, "The Plagues of Egypt," *Zeitschrift fur die Alttestamentliche Wissenschaft* 69 (1957): 84–103.
4. G. Hort, "The Plagues of Egypt. II," *Zeitschrift fur die Alttestamentliche Wissenschaft* 70 (1958): 48–59.
5. J.S. Marr and C.D. Malloy, "An Epidemiologic Analysis of the Ten Plagues of Egypt," *Caduceus* 12, no. 1 (1996): 7–21.
6. G.W. Christopher, et al., "Biological Warfare. A Historical Perspective," *JAMA* 278, no. 5 (1997): 412–417.
7. J.A. Popuard and L.A. Miller, "History of Biological Warfare: Catapults to Capsomeres," *Annals of New York Academy of Sciences* 666 (1992): 9–20.
8. A.G. Robertson and L.J. Robertson, "From Asps to Allegations: Biological Warfare in History," *Military Medicine* 160, no. 8 (1995): 369–373.
9. M.E. Lesho et al., "Feces, Dead Horses, and Fleas. Evolution of the Hostile Use of Biological Agents," *Western Journal of Medicine* 168, no. 6 (1998): 512–516.
10. J.S. Marr and C.D. Malloy, "A Brief History and Inventory of Immunizations," *Journal of Public Health Management and Practice* 2, no. 1 (1996): 82–86.
11. P.D. Blanc, "The Legacy of War Gas," *American Journal of Medicine* 106, no. 6 (1999): 689–690.
12. G. Kolata, *Flu: The Story of the Great Influenza Pandemic of 1918 and the Search for the Virus That Caused It*. New York: Firar, Straus, and Giroux, 1999.
13. S. Harris, "Japanese Biological Warfare Research on Humans: A Case Study of Microbiology and Ethics," *Annals of New York Academy of Sciences* 666 (1992): 21–52.
14. M. Furmanski, "Unlicensed Vaccines and Bioweapon Defense in World War II," *JAMA* 282, no. 9 (1999): 822.
15. A.M. Friedlander, et al., "Anthrax Vaccine: Evidence for Safety and Efficacy against Inhalational Anthrax," *JAMA* 282, no. 22 (1999): 2104–2106.
16. Subcommittee on National Security, Veterans Affairs, and International Relations. United States House of Representatives, *The Department of Defense Anthrax Vaccine Immunization Program: Unproven Force Protection*. Washington, DC: Subcommittee on National Security, Veterans Affairs, and International Relations. United States House of Representatives, 2000.
17. B.J. Bernstein, "The Birth of the U.S. Biological-Warfare Program," *Scientific American* 256, no. 6 (1987): 116–121.
18. E.S. Lazowski and S. Matulewicz, "Serendipitous Discovery of Artificial Positive Weil-Felix Reaction Used in Private Immunological War," *ASM News* 43 (1977): 300–302.
19. "Deception by Immunization," *British Medical Journal* 6089 (1977): 716–717.
20. J.E. Moon, "Biological Warfare Allegations: The Korean War Case," *Annals of New York Academy of Sciences* 666 (1992): 53–83.
21. J.A. Mobley, "Biological Warfare in the Twentieth Century: Lessons from the Past, Challenges for the Future," *Military Medicine* 160, no. 11 (1995): 547–553.
22. C.D. Malloy and J.S. Marr, "Mycotoxins and Public Health: A Review," *Journal of Public Health Management and Practice* 3, no. 3 (1997): 61–69.
23. A. Hay, "A Magic Sword or a Big Itch: An Historical Look at the United States Biological Weapons Programme," *Medicine, Conflict, and Survival* 15, no. 3 (1999): 215–234.
24. A. Hay, "Simulants, Stimulants and Diseases: The Evolution of the United States Biological Warfare Programme, 1945–60," *Medicine, Conflict, and Survival* 15, no. 3 (1999): 198–214.
25. E. Regis. *The Biology of Doom: The History of America's Secret Germ Warfare Project*. New York: Henry Hold and Co., 1999.
26. K. Alibek, *Biohazard: The Chilling True Story of the Largest Covert Biological Weapons Program in the World*. New York: Random House, 1999.
27. N. Press, "Haber's Choice, Hobson's Choice, and Biological Warfare," *Perspectives in Biology and Medicine* 29, no. 1 (1985): 92–108.
28. C.J. Davis, "Nuclear Blindness: An Overview of the Biological Weapons Programs of the Former Soviet Union and Iraq," *Emerging Infectious Diseases* 5, no. 4 (1999): 509–512.
29. M. Meselson, et al., "The Sverdlovsk Anthrax Outbreak of 1979," *Science* 266, no. 5188 (1994): 1202–1208.
30. C.G. Héden, "The 1991 Persian Gulf War: Implications for Biological Arms Control," *Annals of New York Academy of Sciences* 666 (1992): 1–8.
31. R.A. Zilinskas, "Iraq's Biological Weapons. The Past as Future?" *JAMA* 278, no. 5 (1997): 418–424.
32. McNeil Consumer Products Company, Corporate Communication, October 15, 1982.
33. Food and Drug Administration, "Tamper-Evident Packaging Requirements for Over-the-Counter Human Drug Products: FDA. Final Rule," *Federal Register* 63, no. 213 (4 November 1998): 59463–59471.
34. P.E. Dietz, "Dangerous Information: Product Tampering and Poisoning Advice in Revenge and Murder Manuals," *Journal of Forensic Science* 33, no. 5 (September 1988): 1206–1217.
35. T.J. Török, et al., "A Large Community Outbreak of Salmonellosis Caused by Intentional Contamination of Restaurant Salad Bars," *JAMA* 278, no. 5 (1997): 389–395.

36. K.B. Olson, "Aum Shinrikyo: Once and Future Threat?" *Emerging Infectious Diseases* 5, no. 4 (1999): 513–516.
37. S.A. Kolavic, "An Outbreak of Shigella Dysenteriae Type 2 among Laboratory Workers Due to Intentional Food Contamination," *JAMA* 278, no. 5 (1997): 396–398.
38. "Ex-Lab Worker Tainted Food," *The Houston Chronicle*, 12 September 1998, sec. A, p. 48.
39. "The Crazies and Their Poison," *The Economist*, 15 August 1998, sec. 31.
40. V. Kattoulas, "Where Are the Children?" *Newsweek* (16 November 1998): 34–37.
41. M. Asaba, "No Action on Poisonous Situation," *The Daily Yomiuri*, 25 November 1998, sec. A, p. 6.
42. K. Itoi, "Easy Money in Japan," *Newsweek* (21 December 1998): 60–62.
43. R.J. Doyle and N.C. Lee, "Microbes, Warfare, Religion, and Human Institutions," *Canadian Journal of Microbiology* 32, no. 3 (1986): 193–200.
44. W.H. McNeill, *Plagues and Peoples*. New York: Anchor Books/Doubleday, 1998.
45. H. Zinsser, *Rats, Lice and History*. New York: Black Dog & Leventhal Publishers, 1996.

Bioterrorism: A Challenge to Public Health and Medicine

Margaret A. Hamburg

Only a few years ago, an attack with a biological agent would have been considered almost unthinkable. Today, however, the threat of bioterrorism is real and growing. This article will provide a brief overview of the threat of bioterrorism, the special role of public health and medicine, and some of the critical issues that need to be addressed as this nation prepares for this disturbing and potentially catastrophic threat.

ONLY A FEW years ago, an attack with a biological agent would have been considered almost unthinkable. Today, however, the threat of bioterrorism is real and growing. Recent events and emerging intelligence about the interests and activities of certain nations and terrorist or ideological groups suggest that the United States cannot afford to be complacent.[1] This new threat also places a set of pressing demands on public health and medicine to recognize and respond appropriately should such an event occur. In fact, the ability of the public health and medical communities to mobilize rapidly and effectively will be fundamental to the ultimate shape and outcome of a bioterrorist attack. This article will provide a brief overview of the threat of bioterrorism, the special role of public health and medicine, and some of the critical issues that need to be addressed as our nation prepares for this disturbing and potentially catastrophic threat.

The Threat of Biological Terrorism

National security analysts have warned that the United States should expect increasing terrorism in general.[2] Conventional attacks such as bombs remain the most likely mode of terrorism, but there are many reasons to believe that biological agents may be an increasingly attractive approach. Unlike other weapons of mass destruction, pathogens suitable for use as bioweapons can be relatively easy to conceal and easy to release; and depending on the objectives of the terrorist, only a relatively small quantity of material may be needed to cause widespread disease or disruption. Furthermore, information about how to

Margaret A. Hamburg, MD, is Assistant Secretary for Planning and Evaluation for the U.S. Department of Health and Human Services in Washington, DC.

obtain and prepare biological weapons is increasingly available through the Internet and other sources.[3]

New insights into past and possibly ongoing bioweapons-related activities around the world provide further reason for concern about the seriousness of the biological threat. Some examples include: the revelations about the magnitude of the bioweapons program in the former Soviet Union; the disclosure of an ambitious bioweapons program mounted by Iraq; and the findings that Aum Shinrikyo, the Japanese group that released nerve gas in the Tokyo subway, also had experimented with botulism and anthrax and allegedly sent teams to Zaire in an effort to obtain Ebola.[1]

In light of these concerns, many experts now believe that it is no longer a matter of "if" but "when" a bioterrorist attack will occur.[4] Moreover, by its very nature, a biological attack implies a threat that is not limited by geographic boundaries nor is it limited to a discrete event in time. Thus, there is an urgent need to enhance our nation's preparedness and ability to respond to the threat of bioterrorism.

The Nature of Biological Terrorism

It is important to address at the outset the question of why bioterrorism requires public health's specific focus and concern. Clearly, domestic terrorism can involve a range of threats from conventional weapons such as bombs to the so-called weapons of mass destruction, including chemical, nuclear, and biological agents. All of these represent areas of serious concern, but until recently, the almost exclusive focus of counter-terrorism activities has been on models that reflect an explosive, chemical, or nuclear attack. However, the consequence of a bioterrorist attack would be an epidemic and would present a fundamentally distinct set of requirements and challenges. Future preparedness efforts must focus on the prospect of bioterrorism as well.

For example, the 1993 World Trade Center bombing in New York City resulted in colossal damage, substantial terror, numerous injuries, death, and immense disruption in city life as well as enormous economic costs to businesses and the city. Although this bombing incident caused widespread devastation, the silent release of a bioweapon could have created even more havoc.

In such a scenario, thousands of people who were working in that building or visiting would have unknowingly been exposed to a biological agent, returned home, and become ill within days or weeks. With worsening illness, these individuals would begin to come into emergency departments, walk-in clinics, and physicians' offices, but they would be spread out in time and geographic location.

Further compounding the situation would be the fact that many—if not most—of the health care providers who would be seeing the early victims of exposure would not initially recognize the seriousness of the problem and most likely would not identify the disease itself. For example, few physicians in this country have seen a case of smallpox, plague, or anthrax and are unfamiliar with the relevant signs and symptoms. Hence, accurate diagnosis likely would be delayed. Similarly, laboratory capability to rapidly diagnose and type these bio-agents is limited at best. Such delays in diagnosis mean delays in the appropriate implementation of control measures as well as potentially life-saving treatment for those exposed.

Additionally, if the biological agent released was one that produces a communicable disease with person-to-person transmission, and especially if it occurs among travelers, the U.S. would face the possibility of ever-widening circles of exposure, thus extending significantly the damage caused by the terrorist weapon.

Moreover, if the pathogen is smallpox virus or some other organism against which the vast majority of the U.S. population has little or no protective immunity, the resulting devastation would be even greater. In the case of smallpox, for example, this country has not done routine immunization since 1971 and there have been no reported cases of the disease in decades.[5] Similarly, the casualties would escalate dramatically if the pathogen released is one for which no treatment exists either because no effective therapy has been discovered and developed or because the organism has been genetically modified in some way to resist standard therapies.

In reality, a bioterrorist attack could produce an unprecedented public health and medical emergency, rapidly overwhelming the existing health care system at the local level. A potentially large population of people with symptoms of disease would require medical care and treatment and an even larger number of individuals at risk of exposure and disease likely would need preventive care/prophylaxis. Available antibiotics or vaccines would be depleted quickly.

In addition, a bioterrorist event likely would produce severe psychological, behavioral, and social consequences on a scale never experienced before. The prospect of a deadly agent released silently, invisibly, and unpredictably would trigger a level of fear, anxiety, and panic that soon would engulf not just the communities most directly affected but the nation. Mass panic leading to civil disorder and social and economic chaos is a real concern. Such damage to human/social infrastructure can be far more devastating than damage to a physical infrastructure.

For all these reasons, strategies to counter bioterrorism must differ markedly from those applied to terrorism involving other weapons of destruction, whose use is generally immediately obvious and whose effects are confined within an area near the incident site. Clearly, bioterrorism presents a set of serious and unique challenges to the nation's emergency preparedness systems, public health organizations, and medical consequence management capability. However, at this time, the U.S. has a limited array of tools to address these concerns.

Preparing for the Threat of Bioterrorism

Preparedness planning for a bioterrorist threat is critical and challenging. Such planning involves complex issues, substantial uncertainties, and gaps in both our knowledge and capacity. Further, a meaningful and durable response will require effective partnerships among many professional disciplines as well as across all levels of government.

National leadership is essential in defining the nature of the threat and strategies to address it. Indeed, certain elements of the overall response must be provided by the federal government. Many critical policies, programs, and activities must be developed and implemented with federal guidance and support. Later in this article, I will describe some of the actions currently being undertaken by the U.S. Department of Health and Human Services (DHHS)—in collaboration with other federal agencies—to enhance our nation's bioterrorism preparedness and response capability.

Despite the critical need for national leadership and federal guidance, it must be recognized that much of the initial crisis response and subsequent consequence management will unfold on the local level. "On-the-ground" local providers—public health and medical professionals, emergency response personnel, law enforcement officials, and government and community leaders—will provide the foundation of the response and will deal with the problem from the moment the first cases emerge until the crisis is over.

Before such a crisis arises, however, communities must think about the challenges ahead. They should identify and enlist the capabilities and expertise that reside within their communities and work with other communities and across levels of government to understand the constellation of resources that could be available in the event of a crisis. It is now, during a state of relative calm, that public health officials should be building and fostering the relationships across professional disciplines and cultures that will be necessary in working together effectively should a terrorist attack occur.

We urgently need to enhance awareness, strengthen the capability of the public health and medical communities to respond to the threat posed by the major bio-agents, and begin planning and preparing appropriate responses. The U.S. must expand its ability to counter bioterrorism through complementary, simultaneous improvements in the bioterrorism-related expertise, facilities, and procedures at the local, state, and national level including investments in training, preparedness planning, and capacity building.

Elements of an Effective Response

Experts agree that the terrorist use of biological weapons against the civilian population will most likely be surreptitious. As previously discussed, absent an explosion, other immediate evidence of an attack, or notification of authorities by a perpetrator that an attack has occurred, the first responders will be health care providers rather than fire or police personnel as would be expected for a conventional emergency response scenario. The first indication that a silent attack has occurred probably will be an outbreak of some uncommon illness or an abrupt, significant increase in the incidence of commonly observed symptoms such as fever or diarrhea. How quickly the outbreak is detected, analyzed, understood, and addressed will determine the timeliness and effectiveness of the medical and public health response and therefore the extent and severity of the impact on the health and well-being of the affected community. The speed of detection also has important implications for the law enforcement/criminal investigation activities to understand, limit, and prevent future terrorist actions.

Critical to rapid detection will be enhanced disease surveillance systems to ensure an effective response to acts of bioterrorism. We must expand and strengthen our epidemiological capacity to detect and investigate outbreaks as well as new or unusual trends in infectious disease. Correspondingly, laboratory capacity must be sufficient to rapidly analyze and identify biological agents; and the use of electronic communications technology will be essential to quickly collect, analyze, and share information among public health and other officials at local, state, and federal levels. Front-line medical providers must be brought into an increasingly integral partnership with the public health system in order to achieve more effective disease reporting and recognition of unusual clusters or manifestations of illness.

Much of the initial burden and responsibility for effective response to a terrorist attack of any kind rests with the local governments, with supplemental support from state and federal agencies. There is an urgent need to enhance our public health and medical care systems to support medical care for large affected populations, including the development of innovative strategies for delivering both preventive and treatment measures under mass casualty or exposure conditions, especially when there may be a set of very difficult infection control requirements as well. In addition, mass fatality disposition will potentially present significant management and emotional challenges.

The release of a biological weapon also may require rapid access to substantial quantities of pharmaceutical antidotes, antibiotics, or vaccines that would not be readily available in the locations where they were needed. Because no one can anticipate exactly where a terrorist will strike and because such an event is generally low probability but high consequence for any given locality, local communities must have rapid access to critical pharmaceuticals. Yet it would be unrealistic and ill advised to expect communities to use limited resources to create sufficient pharmaceutical stockpiles on their own. The federal government, however, can and should step in to provide the leadership and resources necessary to develop and maintain special stockpiles as a national resource. The Centers for Disease Control and Prevention has been charged with this task and currently is developing plans for both the content and implementation of this national stockpile of pharmaceuticals and related materials to be used to counter epidemics caused by a bioterrorist attack.

Our capability to detect and respond to a bioterrorist attack depends largely on the state of the relevant medical science and technology. Without rapid techniques for accurate identification of pathogens and assessment of their antibiotic sensitivities, planning for the medical and public health response will be compromised significantly. Without efficacious prophylactic and therapeutic agents, even the best-planned responses are likely to fail. Biomedical research is needed to develop new tools for rapid diagnostics, as well as improved drugs and vaccines. The U.S. must invest in research to enhance fundamental understandings of the biological agents likely to be used as weapons of mass destruction as well as in ongoing efforts to better understand the nature of our immune response to different types of infection and the correlates of protective immunity.

In addition to biomedical research, further research into such diverse concerns as defining appropriate personal protective gear or decontamination procedures under different circumstances will be fundamental to our overall preparedness for a bioterrorist attack.

The public health and medical community must also address prevention in terms of measures that can be undertaken to reduce access to dangerous pathogens. Clearly, measures that will deter or prevent bioterrorism will be the most cost-effective means to counter such threats to public health and social order—both in human and economic terms. Are there strategies to limit or prevent these often frightening microbes from getting into the hands of those who might misuse them and how do we reduce the likelihood that they would be misused?

On a policy level, such prevention efforts require a global approach, including the need to support the strengthening and enforcement of the Biological Weapons Convention as well as international scientific cooperation to create opportunities for scientists formerly engaged in bioweapons research to redirect their talents and energy into more constructive and open research arenas. For example, a number of scientific collaborations have begun in Russia in an attempt to address this goal.

We must also strengthen and expand efforts to control access to and handling of certain dangerous pathogens, including proactive measures by the scientific community to monitor more closely the facilities and procedures involved in the use of such biological agents.

DHHS Bioterrorism Initiative

Recognizing this array of pressing concerns and outstanding needs, the DHHS has embarked on a new strategic effort to address the threat of bioterrorism. In fiscal year 1999, for the first time, DHHS received targeted funding ($170 million) specifically for this purpose, and support increased to the level of $285 million in fiscal year 2000. DHHS's activities now focus on five distinct but related areas: (1) deterrence of biological terrorism; (2) public health surveillance; (3) medical and public health response; (4) development of a national pharmaceutical stockpile; and (5) research and development. DHHS hopes to continue to strengthen and expand these efforts in the years to come.

Broader Context of Infectious Disease Threats

These federal efforts are vital to preparing us as a nation ready to respond to such an incident. Many of these activities also are crucial in our efforts to better protect our citizenry against the threat of naturally occurring infectious disease. Indeed, the threat of bioterrorism needs to be considered in the broader context of the public health threat posed by a range of infectious disease concerns.

Although often underappreciated, naturally occurring infectious diseases caused by emerging and reemerging pathogens seriously threaten the health and security of this nation on an ongoing basis. Despite all of the advances in biomedical science, including the explosion of new drugs and vaccines for treating and preventing infectious diseases, the death rate in this country from infectious diseases has, in fact, increased almost 60 percent since 1980.[6] During roughly this same period, dozens of new infectious agents have been discovered—most of them dangerous and many of them deadly. In addition, old diseases such as tuberculosis and rabies have resurged, sometimes in new and more difficult to treat forms because of drug resistance.[7]

Many factors contribute to this changing pattern of infectious disease including shifts in human demographics, improper uses of antibiotics, changes in climate patterns, host-parasite interactions, and microbial evolution. Dramatic expansions in international travel, immigration, and international trade have made it possible for dangerous pathogens to travel faster and further afield as well as spread more easily. In addition, increasing urbanization, changing agricultural practices, and environmental manipulations have altered potential exposures or vectors of disease.

The recent encephalitis outbreak in the New York City region caused by a virus never seen in this hemisphere before—West Nile Virus (WNV)—underscores the nation's continuing vulnerability to new infectious disease threats. It also provides an opportunity for further examination of the current strengths and weaknesses in the nation's ability to detect and respond to an unanticipated biological event, whether naturally occurring or an intentional attack.

During a several-week period beginning in August 1999, 62 known cases of severe disease and seven deaths occurred as a result of WNV. (Personal communication, Marcelle Layton, Assistant Commissioner, Communicable Disease Program, Department of Health, New York.) While unexpected, this outbreak in fact was detected and managed relatively quickly owing to several key factors: an informed and conscientious infectious disease physician in a local hospital who knew to call the New York City Department of Health (NYCDOH) about a possible cluster of unusual disease; a talented team of NYCDOH epidemiologists who rapidly mobilized a broad-based outbreak investigation; and the swift implementation of vector control measures (pesticides, mosquito larval control, and removal of stagnant water). Public education and communication about the nature of the public health problem and the required control measures also were important elements of the response.

Although an initial diagnosis of St. Louis Encephalitis was made in this case based on the epidemiology, serology, and clinical presentation, this soon was changed to WNV after veterinary health professionals identified similar disease in bird populations and further laboratory diagnostics were conducted on both animal and human samples. However, the shift in diagnosis did not require a change in the public health interventions or the medical management of patients.

The significance of this first known appearance of WNV has extended far beyond its meaning for public health and medicine. New York City estimates some $10 million in outbreak management costs alone. Additional economic costs were incurred because of international restrictions on horse and poultry exports from the affected areas.[8] Moreover, it remains to be seen whether this outbreak will represent an isolated event or if the virus will become established and spread in the Western Hemisphere over time.

Whatever the future may hold, the WNV outbreak provides some critical lessons. It offers a vivid illustration of the critical partnership among medical, animal health, and public health professionals in detecting an outbreak, the importance and limitations of laboratory diagnostic capability, the role of public and health care provider education, and the complexity and costs associated with large-scale infectious disease control programs. Dr. Marcelle Layton, NYCDOH Director of Communicable Disease, has noted that "New York City's ability to promptly recognize and respond to this outbreak was in large part due to our planning efforts in recent years for bioterrorism, and illustrates that this preparedness does have dual use for both natural and intentional disease outbreaks."[8(p.6)]

Clearly, from a public health and medical perspective, we must be deeply concerned about the introduction of infectious disease into an unsuspecting U.S. population from natural human, animal, or plant sources as well as from a deliberate or "bioterrorist" action involving the release of a pathogen intended to directly cause disease in the population or to damage the animals, plants, or water supply upon which we depend.

While perhaps still of relatively low probability, the high consequence implications of bioterrorism place it in a special category that requires immediate and comprehensive response. As we move forward to address this disturbing new threat, it is heartening to recognize that the investments we make to strengthen the public health infrastructure for disease surveillance, the investments we make in improved medical consequence management, and the investments we make in basic and clinical research to better understand the nature of infectious diseases, immune response, and the development of new drugs and vaccines all will benefit our efforts to protect the health and safety of the public from both naturally occurring and nefariously introduced infectious disease threats.

REFERENCES

1. D.A. Henderson, "The Looming Threat of Bioterrorism," *Science* 283 (1999): 1279–1282.
2. U.S. Commission on National Security in the 21st Century, "New World Coming: American Security in the 21st Century." Washington, DC, September 15, 1999.
3. R. Danzig and P.B. Berkowsky, "Why Should We Be Concerned about Biological Warfare?" in *Biological Weapons: Limiting the Threat,* ed. J. Lederberg. Cambridge, MA: MIT Press, 1999.
4. D.E. Kaplan. "Terrorism's Next Wave: Nerve Gas and Germs Are the New Weapons of Choice," *U.S. News and World Report* (17 November 1997): 28.
5. D.A. Henderson, et al., "Smallpox as a Biological Weapon: Medical and Public Health Management," *Journal of the American Medical Association* 281, no. 22 (1999): 2127–2136.
6. R.W. Pinner, et al. "Trends in Infectious Diseases Mortality in the United States," *Journal of the American Medical Association* 275, no. 3 (1996): 189–193.
7. U.S. Department of Health and Human Services, Centers for Disease Control and Prevention, *Preventing Emerging Infectious Diseases: A Strategy for the 21st Century.* Atlanta: U.S. Department of Health and Human Services, Centers for Disease Control and Prevention, 1998.
8. M. Schoch-Spana, "A West Nile Virus Post-Mortem," *Biodefense Quarterly* 1, no. 3 (1999): 1–7.

Bioterrorism Preparedness: Planning for the Future

Lisa D. Rotz, Denise Koo, Patrick W. O'Carroll, Richard B. Kellogg, Michael J. Sage, and Scott R. Lillibridge

The release of nerve gas in a Tokyo subway and attempted releases of biological agents by the Aum Shinrikyo cult have demonstrated the willingness and ability of modern-day terrorists to use unconventional weapons. Unlike explosive weapons, the use of biologic weapons may only become apparent once people become ill. The detection and response to these man-made outbreaks will occur initially at the medical and public health levels. Therefore, the Centers for Disease Control and Prevention and its partners are strengthening their response, disease detection, diagnostic, and communication capabilities to better protect the nation's citizens against biological or chemical terrorism.

Introduction

Prior to the bombings of the World Trade Center in New York City and the Alfred P. Murrah Federal Building in Oklahoma City, terrorist activity was perceived as an act of violence that occurred somewhere outside the safe borders of the United States. These attacks, along with the successful release of Sarin gas and the unsuccessful release of biological agents on Tokyo citizens by the doomsday cult, Aum Shinrikyo, served as a wake-up call regarding the potential vulnerability of U.S. civilians to acts of ter-

---

Lisa D. Rotz, MD, *is an infectious diseases trained Medical Epidemiologist with the Bioterrorism Preparedness and Response Program, National Centers for Infectious Diseases, Centers for Disease Control and Prevention (CDC), in Atlanta, Georgia.*

Denise Koo, MD, MPH, *is the Director of the Division of Public Health Surveillance and Informatics, Epidemiology Program Office, CDC, Atlanta, Georgia.*

Patrick W. O'Carroll, MD, *is the Assistant Director for Health Informatics, Public Health Practice Program Office, CDC, Atlanta, Georgia.*

Richard B. Kellogg *is the Laboratory Response Network Interagency Liaison and Coordinator, Bioterrorism Preparedness and Response Program, National Centers for Infectious Diseases, CDC, Atlanta, Georgia.*

Michael J. Sage, MPH, *is the Deputy Director of the Division of Environmental Hazards and Health Effects, National Center for Environmental Health, CDC, Atlanta, Georgia.*

Scott R. Lillibridge, MD, *is the Director of the Bioterrorism Preparedness and Response Program, National Centers for Infectious Diseases, CDC, Atlanta, Georgia.*

rorism.[1,2] In response to this growing concern, the government established the Nunn-Lugar-Domenici Domestic Preparedness Program as a part of the Defense Against Weapons of Mass Destruction (WMD) Act of 1996.[3] This program was intended to enhance federal, state, and local emergency response capabilities to deal with a domestic terrorist incident involving weapons of mass destruction. However, the Nunn-Lugar-Domenici Program did not address the role of public health in responding to acts of terrorism that have the ability to affect large populations.

The pivotal role of public health in addressing the threat of bioterrorism was acknowledged almost 50 years ago by the creation of the U.S. Epidemic Intelligence Service (EIS). This on-the-job epidemiology training program was formed in response to the potential Cold War threat of biological warfare.[4,5] The important role of public health in incidents involving WMD has since been reaffirmed. In 1998, Congress appropriated $158 million to fund an Anti-Bioterrorism Initiative. This Department of Health and Human Services initiative addresses the need for enhanced public health surveillance and laboratory capabilities and a National Pharmaceutical Stockpile to detect, diagnose, and treat illnesses caused by potential bioterrorism pathogens. This initiative will help build the coordinated response and rapid communications across all levels of local, state, and governmental response agencies, which are essential to reducing the consequences of an attack.

The Role of Public Health

Terrorism response training of conventional first responders such as emergency medical technicians, firefighters, and police personnel traditionally has focused on response protocols for explosive devices, firearms, or chemical agents. Such training was appropriately directed at these groups because they are most likely the first ones to arrive at the scene of an explosion or chemical spill. An unannounced dissemination of a biological agent, however, may easily go unnoticed, with the victims leaving the area of the release long before the act of terrorism becomes evident. The first signs that a biological agent has been released probably would not become apparent until days to weeks later, when the victims become ill and present to health care professionals for evaluation. In this type of scenario, it is the health care professional who is considered "first on the scene." An astute physician or nurse very well may provide public health officials with the initial clues that indicate an unannounced or covert biological attack has occurred. Both unannounced and announced attacks with a biological agent would require, among other responses, increased surveillance for illness by both the public health and medical communities as well as rapid implementation of illness prevention measures such as the administration of prophylactic antibiotics or vaccines. To minimize the adverse health consequences of bioterrorism, public health officials must act quickly to detect and respond effectively to such events as well as to assist the medical community in its preparedness and response efforts.

There are five components to a comprehensive public health response to a naturally occurring outbreak of illness: (1) detecting the outbreak, (2) determining the cause of the illness, (3) identifying factors that place people at risk for illness, (4) implementing measures to control the outbreak, and (5) informing the medical and public communities about treatments, health consequences, and preventive measures. The components of a public health response to biological terrorism are essentially the same. However, a public health system already pressed with routine public health activities will quickly become overtaxed with the enormous response necessary in a bioterrorist event as will a health care delivery system that maintains a limited ability to operate at excess capacity.

Focus Areas for Future Preparedness

Preparing the nation to address the threat of bioterrorism is a major challenge to our public health and health care systems. The early detection needed to minimize the morbidity and mortality associated with the potentially lethal agents of bioterrorism requires increased awareness among members of the medical community and improved linkages between both the medical and public health communities on local, state, and federal levels. Local and state health agencies require the necessary epidemiological capacity and expertise to detect and investigate rapidly any unusual and unexplained illnesses. In addition, diagnostic laboratories must have specially trained personnel and the appropriate equipment to identify biological and chemical agents that rarely are encountered in the United States.

Because a biological terrorist attack can take place covertly, an outbreak of an unknown illness may be the first indicator of such an attack. The Centers for Disease Control and Prevention (CDC) currently is enhancing public health capabilities to address unknown illnesses with the implementation of a strategic plan for the prevention of new and emerging infectious diseases.[6] The improved capabilities to detect and respond to natural outbreaks caused by new or emerging pathogens also will enhance capabilities to detect and respond to potential bioterrorism pathogens, many of which can cause rare and unusual diseases that are difficult to diagnose. In addition, to further prepare public health for detecting and rapidly responding to acts of biological and chemical terrorism, the CDC has focused on enhancing five key areas: (1) preparedness and readiness assessment, (2) detection and surveillance, (3) identification and characterization of biological and chemical agents, (4) response, and (5) information and communications.

Preparing for and responding to bioterrorism will be a complex process involving the activities of many local, state, and federal agencies. In order to mitigate the consequences of an attack, coordinated preparedness efforts at the local, state, and federal level are essential to ensure a well-organized and routinely tested response plan. In addition to improving its own preparedness and response capabilities, the CDC is developing public health guidelines and providing support and technical assistance to state and local public health partners as they develop bioterrorism preparedness plans and response protocols. To assist these partners in evaluating these plans, the CDC is developing self-assessment tools for preparedness including performance standards, proficiency testing programs, attack simulations, and other response exercise materials. The CDC also encourages and supports applied research to develop innovative tools and strategies such as computerized resource tracking systems to prevent or minimize the overall consequences of bioterrorism. To fund these efforts, the CDC awarded approximately $1.5 million to nine states and two cities in 1999, with plans to award funding for preparedness and response efforts in additional states during the next 3–5 years.

Early detection of a bioterrorist event by enhanced surveillance is essential because it can lead to a quick response. A timely public health response would prevent illness by ensuring that prophylactic medications or vaccines are administered to those who were exposed but not yet ill as well as facilitate the rapid diagnosis and treatment of those who are already ill. With its state and local public health partners, the CDC is integrating surveillance for illness and injury from potential biological or chemical agents into the nation's disease surveillance systems. Novel mechanisms, such as syndromic-based or hospital admission surveillance systems, and Internet-based reporting currently are being developed and evaluated for their usefulness in detecting and rapidly reporting suspicious adverse health events that might represent a covert terrorist attack. In addition, the CDC and its public health partners continue to explore new alliances and joint educational efforts with front-line medical partners such as hospital emergency departments, professional medical organizations, poison control centers, and emergency medical services to further enhance the recognition and reporting of unexplained injuries and illnesses. To improve state and local surveillance capabilities, the CDC awarded more than $7.8 million to 31 states and three large cities in 1999. During the next several years, funds awarded to additional states will serve to further enhance public health surveillance efforts.

Many of the potential bioterrorism agents cause rare (e.g., inhalational anthrax, pneumonic plague) or even previously globally eradicated diseases (e.g., smallpox), making them a less likely consideration in the differential diagnosis of an illness. Rapid identification and characterization of the biological or chemical agent used in a bioterrorist attack ensure that the correct prophylactic, therapeutic, and control measures are instituted. Isolating and identifying these agents pose a substantial challenge to the current public health and medical laboratory systems because most laboratories do not possess the clinical awareness and advanced technology to identify these agents rapidly. The CDC and its public health partners are establishing a multi-level Laboratory Response Network for Bioterrorism, which ultimately will link public health agencies from 50 states, nine territories, and several additional counties and cities to advanced-capacity referral facilities. These referral facilities will maintain state-of-the-art diagnostic capabilities for a wide range of biological agents.

The CDC has awarded a total of almost $8.8 million in grants to 41 state and two large city health laboratories to upgrade their diagnostic capabilities for biological critical agents. In addition, the CDC has awarded $4 million in funds and transferred sophisticated instrumentation and diagnostic technology to four select state health laboratories to upgrade their capabilities to diagnose human illness from chemical exposures and to establish a regional Chemical Terrorism Laboratory Network. This network would provide diagnostic overflow capacity to the CDC for large chemical events. To enhance internal rapid diagnostic capabilities for biological threat agents, the CDC has also created an internal Rapid Response and Advanced Technology Laboratory to provide 24-hour diagnostic support for national and international outbreaks of unknown illnesses possibly caused by bioterrorism.

The public health response to bioterrorism will involve a rapid epidemiological investigation, medical treatment and prophylaxis of affected individuals, and the institution of disease prevention or environmental control measures. The CDC assists state and local health agencies in strengthening their resources and expertise to investigate unusual adverse health events and unexplained illnesses. Additional personnel are being recruited into the EIS training program and bioterrorism-directed training is being integrated into the EIS two-year curriculum. The CDC can also deploy a specialized epidemiological and laboratory response team to assist in the investigation of unexplained or suspicious outbreaks of illness and provide on-site consultation on medical management and disease control measures at the request of state health departments. In addition, the CDC was allocated $51 million in 1999 to create a National Pharmaceutical Stockpile to ensure the availability of medical therapeutics and equipment necessary to treat illness from biological and chemical terrorism agents. The agency plans to spend additional funds to augment this stockpile in future years.

Rapid and reliable communication between public health agencies at all levels is essential both for preparedness efforts and for the coordination of a response to an actual event. The ability to disseminate and share information rapidly among public health officials during a bioterrorist event ensures that all decisions are made with the most current information available. Effective communication with the media and public functions to minimize public panic and ensure the reliable dissemination of essential information on signs of illness, treatment, and control measures.

The CDC is working with state and local health agencies to build the Health Alert Network (HAN), a national telecommunications and distance-learning network that will provide all full-function local public health agencies with (1) high-capacity, continuous Internet connections for secure electronic communications and Web access; (2) the capacity to receive satellite- or Web-based distance learning on bioterrorism and other health threats; (3) the capacity to send targeted health alerts to various community subgroups (e.g., hospital medical staff) through broadcast fax or other broadcast technologies; and (4) the guidance by which to measure their organization's capacity to detect and respond to bioterrorism and other health threats. The CDC distributed almost $19 million in 1999 to 33 state and three large city health departments for the development of HAN. Additional states will receive funding during the next several years.

Outcomes of Preparedness

As the national disease control and prevention agency, the CDC must ensure that the U.S. public health system is capable of mounting a prompt and effective response to bioterrorism. With the successful implementation of these preparedness activities during the next several years, the U.S. public health and medical systems will be better prepared to mitigate the consequences of a biological or chemical terrorist event. Enhanced epidemiological, surveillance, laboratory, and communication capabilities will not only ensure an effective and coordinated response to such attacks but also will strengthen the ability to detect and respond to non-bioterrorist outbreaks. This fortification of the nation's overall public health infrastructure in response to the threat of bioterrorism ultimately will serve to better protect the nation against all threats to its health.

REFERENCES

1. T. Okumura, et al., "The Tokyo Subway Sarin Attack: Disaster Management, Part 1: Community Emergency Response," *Academy of Emergency Medicine* 5, no. 6 (1998): 613–617.
2. K.B. Olson, "Aum Shinrikyo: Once and Future Threat?" *Emerging Infectious Diseases* 5, no. 4 (1999): 513–516.
3. The Defense Against Weapons of Mass Destruction Act. The National Defense Authorization Act for Fiscal Year 1997; Title XIV of P.L. (1996).
4. A.D. Langmuir and J.M. Andrews, "Biological Warfare Defense. 2. The Epidemic Intelligence Service of the Communicable Disease Center," *American Journal of Public Health* 42 (1952): 235–238.
5. S.B. Thacker, et al., "Training and Service in Public Health Practice, 1951–90-CDC's Epidemic Intelligence Service," *Public Health Reports* 105 (1990): 599–604.
6. Centers for Disease Control and Prevention, *Preventing Emerging Infectious Diseases: A Strategy for the 21st Century.* Atlanta: U.S. Department of Health and Humans Services, 1998.

Intergovernmental Preparedness and Response to Potential Catastrophic Biological Terrorism

Steven Kuhr and Jerome M. Hauer

The 20th century is replete with examples of the use of biological weapons in times of war. Today, it is only a matter of time before terrorists find a way to develop and deploy biological weapons as well. Because of the narrow window of opportunity in which treatment and prophylaxis can positively affect the outcome of those exposed to and infected by biological weapons, aggressive public health surveillance is the best early defense. A casualty management and mass prophylaxis campaign will require coordination at all levels of government involving many agencies.

Introduction

On March 20, 1995, the world had an opportunity to watch the response to catastrophic terrorism from their living rooms. Aum Shinrikyo (Supreme Truth), a Japanese-based cult with international interests, released the chemical nerve agent Sarin into the Tokyo subway system, killing 12 commuters and injuring some 5,000 others. Some would say that this incident was the catalyst that brought international attention to the reality of terrorism using weapons of mass injury and death by terrorist organizations.

Weapons capable of causing mass injury, illness, and death have marked their place in the history of the 20th century. Although most of this history is related to the use of these agents during times of war, the efficiency of these weapons has not gone unnoticed by terrorists. Aum Shinrikyo made several attempts to weaponize and release biological agents including *clostridium botulinum* and *bacillus anthracis.*[1] (Personal communication, K. Olson, Project Manager, Research Planning, Inco, November 5, 1999.) In another incident in 1984, the followers of the Rajneesh, the leader of a cult based in Oregon, sprayed *salmonella typhimurium* bacteria on open salad bars in a number of restaurants throughout the city of The Dalles, Oregon. About 750 people were

__Steven Kuhr__ is a Managing Director at the Strategic Emergency Group, Ltd., in East Northport, New York.

__Jerome M. Hauer, MHS__, was formerly Director of the Mayor's Office of Emergency Management in New York, New York. He is currently Assistant Vice President and Associate Director of the Science Applications International Corporation Center for Counterterrorism Technology and Analysis.

sickened; no deaths were recorded.[2–4] These attacks illustrate that terrorists recognize the potential of biological agents as weapons, which can have even greater consequences than chemical agents. While the use of biological weapons by terrorists has been limited, it is clearly only a matter of time until an incident of mass biological terrorism is visited on an unsuspecting city.

Analysis and Preparedness

In order for governments to prepare for efficient response to biological terrorism, an introspective analysis of local, regional, and national programs serves as a good first step in identifying strengths and weaknesses in systems designed to recognize and respond to unusual and exotic disease outbreaks. Preparedness and response programs are not the unique domain of any one particular agency or organization. This is especially true in the public health and medical communities where a close relationship is needed to closely coordinate and integrate planning and preparedness initiatives.

Planning for bioterrorism can be broken down into modular components, each of which serves as a building block in the structure of an entire program. These building blocks require multi-agency involvement and include:

- surveillance and recognition
- epidemiology and investigation
- mass prophylaxis
- casualty and fatality management
- logistical coordination
- exercise design and evaluation

Surveillance and Recognition

Surveillance is needed at the regional level if early recognition of a biological terrorism incident will occur. This is essential in metropolitan areas where cities share populations. New York City, for example, shares a population of 12 million with the surrounding suburban areas. While eight million reside within the city limits, an additional four million commute to the city every workday. Add in thousands of tourists who visit the city every day and one gets a sense of the enormity of the population. When considering the potential for an incident to occur in a city, with the effects being transmitted throughout the surrounding suburban communities, the need for regional surveillance is clear; enter the issue of interagency, interjurisdictional, and intergovernmental coordination.

Emergency management agencies (EMAs), by their very nature, are coordinating bodies of governments at the local, state, and federal levels. Closely aligned, especially for planning and response to terrorism, are public health agencies that, by their very nature, monitor, conduct investigations, and respond to unusual disease outbreaks. Partnerships between EMAs and public health agencies are emerging daily as the threat of biological terrorism is recognized as a major issue to confront. The need for this partnership is highlighted when integrating health surveillance systems; coordination will be critical if surveillance systems will be regionalized. While emergency management and public health agencies serve as the nexus of health surveillance and response, many other agencies and health care organizations can contribute to surveillance programs.

Emergency medical service

Emergency medical service (EMS), the gateway to health care for many, especially in dense urban areas, is an important partner in bioterrorism planning. EMS activity serves as a good barometer to gauge the health of a population. In general, EMS activity increases when unusual disease patterns emerge. This is evident especially during annual influenza season. Other environmental conditions also affect EMS activity including extremes of cold and heat and foul weather. When a baseline is developed for normal EMS run patterns, including an analysis and understanding of EMS service demand during periods of peak use (such as influenza season or heat wave events), a surveillance system can be implemented. Surveillance can be conducted daily or even hourly to identify unusual elevations of demand that might be an early indication of an emerging health crisis (clearly the benefit of this goes beyond bioterrorism as disease monitoring in general is enhanced as well).

Hospitals

Hospital emergency department (ED) activity also serves as an excellent tool when gauging the health of a community. Many bioterrorism agents present with an influenza-like syndrome. As the disease process progresses, people seeking health care will flood the offices of their primary care physicians as well as EDs (consider also that some of the ED volume will arrive through EMS transport). Capturing and monitoring these data, locally and regionally, also are essential if early recognition of an incident were to occur. Once the system to monitor general ED and admission data is developed and takes hold, assessing data on specific syndromes, such as respiratory illness and fevers of unknown origin, can strengthen the surveillance program.

Medical examiners

Local medical examiners and coroners play a critical role in health surveillance as well. Medical examiner data offer additional insight into the health of a population. Analyzing trends in deaths in a community and developing a baseline against which one can gauge daily death statistics allows for a quick identification of spikes that may be indicative of an emerging disease outbreak.

Centralized data capture

The key here is centralization of data capture for purposes of cataloguing the data and monitoring for unusual trends. This strengthens the ability to make a daily analysis from a single source. The Office of Emergency Management (OEM) in New York City serves as this clearinghouse. Each day at 7 AM, the Fire Department–EMS, Health and Hospitals Corporation, and Office of the Chief Medical Examiner report their data for the preceding 24-hour period to OEM communications. The data then are consolidated into a single report, which is provided to senior emergency management and public health officials. As mentioned above, the data sets include Fire Department–EMS demand, hospital activity for a dozen sentinel hospitals throughout the city, and medical examiner data that include total reported deaths as well as deaths accepted for further investigation and autopsy. These data then are measured against the baseline as well as environmental conditions such as temperature, humidity, heat index, or wind chill.

Reporting

Most public health departments also require physicians and other medical personnel to report unusual infectious and contagious diseases. Eight biological agents (see Table 1) exist that should appear on every local list as a reportable disease. The reporting requirement also should include that a notification be made upon recognition or suspicion of any unusual or exotic disease. This will allow public health officials to gather information from as many sources as possible. Reporting emerging diseases must become routine; it is the responsibility of public health agencies to ensure that medical practitioners are instructed to make timely notifications. Conversely, public health agencies also must alert medical practitioners of emerging disease events as they become aware of them. This will alert medical personnel and hopefully raise their awareness and index of suspicion.

Epidemiology and Investigation

If after reviewing the data generated by the health surveillance system, it is believed that an outbreak is occurring, public health officials can then embark on an epidemiological investigation in an attempt to identify the disease and perhaps even the source. This investigation should take a regional focus in order to identify the agent as quickly as possible if it is determined that a biological attack has occurred (with proper planning, this can be conducted in coordination with law enforcement officials). A narrow window of opportunity exists to begin medical care and mass prophylaxis; time is of the essence. Consider the release of a military grade bacterial agent in a commuter rail station. Thousands of people from various communities in and around a metropolitan area could potentially become victims of this attack. Involving public health and EMAs in all these areas will lead to a rapid and organized response. Intergovernmental and interagency coordination is critical. State public health departments are in the best position to coordinate a regional epidemiological investigation, especially where multiple jurisdictions are involved. The U.S. Public Health Service also will have a role if the metropolitan region includes another state or multiple states.

Mass Prophylaxis

After a biological terrorist incident has been recognized, the clock is ticking. This is especially true when dealing with bacterial agents where treatment

Table 1

Reportable biological agents

Agent	Disease	Classification	Incubation period	Treatment	Optimal time to begin treatment
Bacillus anthracis	Anthrax	Bacteria	1–5 days	Ciprofloxacin Doxycycline Penicillin	24 hours: When symptoms appear from aerosol exposure, expect high mortality rates
Francisella tularensis	Tularemia	Bacteria	1–10 days	Streptomycin Doxycycline	Antibiotic therapy should begin upon disease suspicion
Coxiella burnetii	Q-fever	Bacteria	14–26 days	Tetracycline Doxycycline	Antibiotic therapy should begin late in the incubation period, advanced epidemiology needed
Brucella species	Brucellosis	Bacteria	5–21 days	Streptomycin Tetracycline	Antibiotic therapy should begin upon disease suspicion and may need to be continued for six weeks
Yersinia pestis	Plague (contagious)	Bacteria	1–3 days	Ciprofloxacin Doxycycline Streptomycin	Antibiotic therapy should begin upon disease suspicion and should continue for 3–4 days after clinical recovery
Variola	Smallpox (contagious)	Virus	10–12 days	Supportive care	Antiviral agent not available
Venezuolan equine encephalitis virus	Venezuelan equine encephalitis	Virus	1–6 days	Supportive care	Antiviral agent not available
Staphylococcus Enterotoxin (B)	Intoxication	Toxin	1–6 hours	Supportive care	Antitoxin not available

Source: Data from F. Sidell, W. Patrick, and T. Dashiell. *Jane's Chem-Bio Handbook.* Jane's Information Group, Alexandria, Virginia, 1998; *Textbook of Military Medicine: Medical Aspects of Chemical and Biological Warfare.* Office of the Surgeon General, United States Army, 1997.

and prophylaxis with antibiotics can positively affect the outcomes of those exposed and infected. Anthrax is probably the best example of why mass treatment and prophylaxis must be instituted immediately. When a victim begins showing signs and symptoms of anthrax infection, it is questionable whether antibiotics will have any effect. Two models to prophylax the population have been examined: (1) bringing the medications to the people or (2) bringing the people to the medications. Bringing medications to the people is extremely resource intensive and will require the activation of thousands of individuals such as the National Guard and military to deliver thousand of doses of antibiotics within the timeframe required to treat and avoid illness. On the other hand, bringing people to the medications requires fewer resources. This method requires the establishment of medication distribution centers in affected communities. Through mass media, aggressive community outreach, and other sources such as the Internet, people are instructed on where to report for their medications. These facilities can be established in community centers, local sports stadiums and ball fields, theaters, or any location that can handle the mass influx of people.

Casualty and Fatality Management

Caring for the sick and dying will be another huge undertaking. Hospitals and EMS systems may be overwhelmed to a level never before experienced. Augmenting the health care system will be a major priority in order to treat as many people in as short a time as possible. Hospitals will have to supplement their capabilities internally by commissioning decommissioned beds and by establishing care areas in space never used before for patient care. This might include cafeterias and other open spaces.

Concurrently, the government's medical response should include the establishment of alternate care centers near hospitals to relieve them of some of the patient load as well as casualty collection points, which essentially are hospitals established in areas where none currently exist. As people succumb to the disease, fatality management will be a critical issue. Proper and timely disposal of the deceased will have to be a coordinated effort among the medical examiner, public health department, and law enforcement agencies, which may consider each body as evidence.

Logistical Coordination

Coordinated movement of materials and human resources to support the mass prophylaxis and casualty management operation will be yet another large and essential component of the response. As materials such as medications and medical supplies arrive, they will have to be catalogued and deployed to locations based on prioritized need. Pre-planning for this will have long-term benefits. This might include identifying a specific hangar at an airport where federal assets can arrive as well as pre-designating transportation from the airport to hospitals and casualty collection points.

This effort will require the integration and cooperation of many agencies. Table 2 shows the agencies and functions for a biological weapon attack on a typical American city. Myriad other agencies exist at all levels of government; however, their role in terrorism response is outside the scope of this article.

Bringing It All Together: Exercise Design and Evaluation

Executing a response for a catastrophic bioweapons attack would be an operation never before seen in this country. In order to ensure that the response occurs as expected, exercises are required to challenge the agencies at all levels of government. These include table-top scenarios where agencies are brought together in a nonstressful environment and given a set of circumstances for which they are asked to respond. Agencies then engage in a facilitated dialogue where they discuss their response. The facilitators then bring up points for discussion such as response obstacles and operational deficiencies. Table-top exercises often are followed up with exercises that are then conducted in a more stressful, real-time environment. This allows the agencies to gauge their response at varying levels of intensity. They can then make the necessary modifications and enhancements to their emergency operations plans.

■ ■ ■

While little experience in dealing with biological terrorism exists, it is clear that the threat must be confronted. Rogue nations are known to possess biological weapons in their arsenals and given the right amount of time, training, and funding, terrorists will gain the knowledge and tools needed to produce biological agents as well. The public health community is the front line of defense against bioterrorism. Enhancing public health and emergency management programs to include preparedness initiatives focused directly on bioweapons surveillance and detection can make all the difference in commencing an early response.

Table 2

Agency response to bioterrorism

Local agencies	Function
Local public health	Health surveillance; epidemiological investigation; patient care protocols; communication with medical community
Local emergency management	Monitor health surveillance data in coordination with the public health department; interagency coordination—emergency operations center (EOC) management; coordinate logistical operations; coordinate with regional, state, and federal agencies including requests for federal and state disaster and terrorism response assets and requests for federal disaster assistance; deploy federal and state assets such as National Guard teams, Disaster Medical Assistant Teams (DMATs), Disaster Mortuary Teams (DMORTs), and military units in coordination with public health, hospitals, and medical examiner
Local law enforcement	Criminal investigation in coordination with FBI; security and crowd control at medication distribution centers, alternate care centers, casualty collection points, hospitals, and pharmacies; security and escort of medical personnel and medical materials including, and especially, antibiotics
Local EMS	Monitor run volume for general increases and increases in specific syndromes such as influenza-like illness, respiratory illness, and fevers of unknown origin; augment service capabilities by increasing staffing and rolling stock if available; activate mutual aid plans to ensure continued emergency service to the affected communities and the general public
Local hospitals	Augment internal patient care capabilities; increase staffing; inventory and ensure adequate supplies of medications and medical materials; coordinate patient care with public health department; coordinate requests for assistance and resources through emergency management—EOC
Local fire service	Support EMS activities; evaluate and ensure fire safety at medication distribution centers, alternate care centers and casualty collection points; support logistical activities with manpower and vehicles; provide resources as requested by emergency management—EOC; deploy HAZMAT team to sites identified as the potential source of the release
Local medical examiner	Implement enhanced capabilities for storing and disposing of mass fatalities including infected remains (refrigerated trailers and rail box cars); activate alternate morgue facilities; integrate Federal DMORTs
Local general services agency	Coordinate closely with emergency management—EOC; ensure that adequate quantities of medical supplies and other materials are available; maintain running log of expenses

State agencies	Function
State public health	Coordinate health surveillance and monitoring over multiple jurisdictions; coordinate epidemiological investigation involving multiple local health agencies; communicate medical matters to hospitals and private practitioners throughout the region and the state; coordinate requests for medical personnel and materials in support of local hospitals; provide laboratory services
State emergency management	Coordinate and execute a response for requests for state and federal assets and disaster assistance; coordinate the response of all state agencies through the state EOC
National Guard	Provide logistical support to move materials and personnel; deploy, if requested, MSD RAID teams (National Guard-based chemical/biological response teams)
State law enforcement	Coordinate closely with local law enforcement and FBI on matters pertaining to the criminal investigation; ensure traffic patterns allow access to city for incoming disaster assistance assets
State EMS	Coordinate mutual aid in the affected region; ensure that local EMS agencies have the resources necessary to maintain adequate response coverage for the affected community as well as the general public
State fire service	Coordinate the delivery of mutual aid with the local fire service; ensure that the local fire service has adequate resources to provide fire/rescue service to the affected and unaffected communities

continues

Table 2

Continued

Federal agencies	Function
FBI	Serve as lead federal agency for crisis management (law enforcement matters); establish a Joint Operations Center (JOC) to coordinate the federal response during the early states of the incident
FEMA	Serve as lead federal agency for consequence management (dealing with actual response to the incident); serve as overall lead federal agency when the crisis phase has been secured; coordinate the response of all federal agencies through the Federal Response Plan; deploy an Emergency Response Team (ERT) to the local EOC early in the incident to determine, with local and state authorities, the needs of the federal response; establish a Regional Operations Center (ROC) to coordinate the federal response; establish a National EOC to coordinate the national response in support of the local jurisdiction or region
U.S. Public Health Service	Serve as the coordinating federal agency for the federal medical response; activate and deploy federal medical assets including those falling under the National Disaster Medical System (NDMS); DMAT, National Medical Response Teams (NMRTs), DMORTs, and medical assets from the DoD, VA, and more as needed
CDC	Coordinate the national pharmaceutical stockpile (antibiotics and medical materials); provide expertise in infectious disease management; provide laboratory support
DoD (Joint Forces Command–Joint Task Force–Civil Support)	Provide medical assets at the request of FEMA and the U.S. Public Health Service; provide logistical movement of federal assets under NDMS; provide specialized U.S. Army and Marine Corps response teams; provide laboratory, infectious disease, and biological terrorism agent expertise from the U.S. Army Institute for Infectious Diseases (USAMRIID) and the Naval Medical Research Institute (NMRI)

REFERENCES

1. K. Olson, Executive Briefing at the Mayor's Office of Emergency Management, New York City, January 12, 1999.
2. T.J. Torok, et al., "A Large Community Outbreak of Salmonellosis Caused by Intentional Contamination of Restaurant Salad Bars," *JAMA* 278, no. 5 (1997):389–395.
3. Federal Bureau of Investigation, "Excerpts: FBI Report on Domestic Terrorism (Domestic Terrorism Shifts to the Right)." http://www.usis-israel.org.il/publish/press/justice/archive/1997/april/jd10418.htm. (17 April 1997). Accessed April 18, 2000.
4. WBFF staff, "Food Terrorism." http://www.wbff45.com/news/97/ft.htm. Accessed April 18, 2000.

Bioterrorism: Challenges and Opportunities for Local Health Departments

Richard J. Gallo and Dyan Campbell

The emerging threat of bioterrorism will significantly impact local health departments. If a bioterrorism attack occurs, local medical and public health personnel will have the primary role of recognition and response. Federal assistance and training to deal with bioterrorism have been directed to 120 of our largest cities. Despite progress, much needs to be done. The public health approach to bioterrorism must begin with the development of local and state plans developed by public health, emergency response, and law enforcement communities, which must work together closely if an epidemic is to be detected in a timely manner.

UNTIL RECENTLY, bioterrorism was not actively discussed or addressed as a concern by local health officials. The focus of most local health departments has been on maintaining existing surveillance systems and disease control programs and finding the resources to deal with new and reemerging diseases. The increasing concern over the emerging threat of bioterrorism is impacting local health departments significantly. Public officials are faced with the challenge of preparing for the possibility of an intentional release of infectious agents upon the people in their jurisdictions.

When confronted with terrorist threats and acts within the United States, it is almost always local authorities who must address the initial response. It is their efforts in the minutes following a terrorist act that will save lives, contain the scope of the crisis, and apprehend terrorists who may be fleeing the scene.[1] In the past, these terrorist acts, with few exceptions, have been carried out with the use of conventional explosives. The first responders have been emergency medical services, fire, rescue, and police personnel.

The authors gratefully acknowledge Robert G. Westphal, MD for his valuable comments on this article. They also thank Quinten Williams for his clerical help in the preparation of this article.

***Richard J. Gallo** is a Community Health Program Manager for the New York State Department of Health in New Rochelle, New York.*

***Dyan Campbell, BN, RN, MPH,** was the Director for the Sullivan County Public Health Nursing Service in Liberty, New York, until retiring in December 1999.*

In the event of an unannounced bioterrorist attack, the entire setting and response changes. A bioterrorist attack may be difficult to distinguish from a naturally occurring infectious disease outbreak. Biological agents have incubation periods; affected persons may not have symptoms for days or weeks after the attack. It will be medical and public health personnel, not fire or law enforcement, who will be the "first responders." Physicians in emergency departments or physician's offices must recognize and report cases. Public health personnel must be able to recognize patterns of infections and conduct epidemiological investigations to establish the likely time and place of exposure as well as the population at risk and the mode of transmissions. Laboratory personnel either in the private or public setting must be able to rapidly identify the infectious agent.

One could take the overly optimistic approach and say that with the interest in bioterrorism comes much-needed federal funding for improved surveillance and response. Funding for bioterrorism preparedness will not only improve our ability to effectively respond to the threat or consequence of a bioterrorism attack but it also will improve our ability to respond to naturally occurring infectious diseases by strengthening state and local public health infrastructure and surveillance systems.

The Defense Against Weapons of Mass Destruction Act of 1996, enacted as the Nunn-Lugar-Domenici Amendment (Nunn-Lugar II) to the Department of Defense Appropriations Act for fiscal year (FY) 1997, mandates that the Executive Branch of the U.S. government undertake a number of requirements relating to preparedness to respond to terrorist use of chemical and biological weapons within the U.S. Among other things, the legislation requires the Executive Branch to assess its capabilities to assist state and local governments in preventing and responding to terrorist incidents involving such weapons.[1] The Domestic Preparedness Program formed under this legislation received about $52 million in FY 1997, and President Clinton asked for $49.5 million in FY 1998 and $52 million in FY 1999 to continue to provide emergency response, first responder training, and assistance to metropolitan area agencies as well as to conduct exercises and preparedness tests in coordination with federal, state, and local agencies.[2]

The program was inspired partly by three deadly terrorist attacks: (1) the 1993 bombing and attempted chemical attack on the New York World Trade Center, (2) the 1995 Aum Shinrikyo "doomsday cult" Sarin gas attack on the Tokyo subway system, and (3) the 1995 bombing of the Alfred P. Murrah Federal Building in Oklahoma City.[3] In addition, Iraq used chemical weapons on Iran as well as on its own citizens and appears to have concealed a biological weapons program.[4] To date, federal assistance and training have been directed to 120 of our nation's largest cities. Despite progress, much needs to be done, particularly in medical and laboratory preparedness, communications, response coordination, and training of key personnel outside of the major urban centers.

Many of the 120 cities receiving federal support are well on their way to having coordinated plans involving local, state, and federal agencies in combating bioterrorism threats and the consequences of a bioterrorist attack. Carrying out these plans presents a number of important challenges.

Assessing the Threat

The potential spectrum of bioterrorism ranges from hoaxes and the use of non-mass casualty devices and agents by individuals or small groups to state-sponsored terrorism that employs classic biological warfare agents and can produce mass casualties.[5]

The nation's large metropolitan areas are the most likely targets for large-scale terrorist attacks, and it is logical to concentrate our training and planning efforts in the largest cities; but other communities remain vulnerable and likely will be involved in the response to any large-scale event.

A successful bioterrorist attack would affect people beyond a city's borders because of potential downwind airborne spread of an infectious agent to surrounding areas. In addition, many of the nation's cities have large numbers of commuters that live in surrounding and more distant counties or states. When exposed to a bioterrorist attack, these commuters could become ill at their homes rather than at their work sites and could tax the resources of their communities significantly.

Domestic bioterrorism could occur anywhere in the United States. The most significant act of bioterrorism to occur in the United States was the intentional contamination of 10 salad bars with *salmonella typhimurium* by the Rajneesh cult in 1984. The event occurred in and around the town of The Dalles, Oregon (population 11,060) and resulted in 751 cases of food poisoning.[6] Although intentional contamination was considered a possibility by public health investigators, the deliberate nature of the outbreak was not confirmed until a separate criminal investigation was conducted. Local police, rescue, medical, and public health workers should be trained to recognize suspicious events and to respond accordingly if a natural or intentional exposure to biological agents occurs.

Where necessary, local public health officials should educate their elected officials about the threat of bioterrorism and request that a response to threats and acts of bioterrorism be incorporated into existing emergency response plans. In addition, each local health department has the opportunity and responsibility to educate its citizens about the threat of bioterrorism. If an attack or incident occurs, it will become a local large-scale emergency.

Planning for Bioterrorism

The public health approach to bioterrorism must begin with the development of local and state plans formulated collaboratively by public health, emergency response, and law enforcement communities, who must work together closely if an epidemic is to be detected in a timely manner.[7]

The Federal Bureau of Investigation (FBI) is the federal agency responsible for investigating all terrorist threats and acts within the United States. The FBI will conduct a criminal investigation concurrent with local public health and the local medical community's response. These efforts will require a coordinated response.[1]

Depending on the level of the incident, other federal and regional agencies like the Federal Emergency Management Agency, the Department of Defense, the Centers for Disease Control and Prevention, and the Department of Agriculture may be called in. Unlike a physical attack, such as a bombing, an announced or covert biological attack does not have a defined time or area, and it is often difficult and time consuming to trace and identify the source or origin. There is a need for planning for mass medical care including mass prophylaxis and mortuary care. There needs to be a local and regional inventory of resources already in place; for example, hospital beds, ventilators, staff, available shelters, and some plan and process of deployment and sharing that transcends county, state, and country borders. A bridge between emergency preparedness and disease outbreak efforts needs to be developed. There will be mental health issues and a need for counseling support to mobilize after a threat or attack. There may be animal or vector control issues as well as an evaluation of whether or not there has been food or water contamination. It is incumbent on public health leaders to replace complacency with a sense of urgency.

The recent emergence of the West Nile Virus in New York City in August 1999 is an example of a naturally occurring outbreak that was controlled after incorporating the same elements of response necessary to contend with a bioterrorism emergency. It involved the initial identification of unusual cases of encephalitis by the medical community, surveillance and control by local public health departments, ruling out bioterrorism by the FBI, laboratory and technical support at the state, federal, and military level, and a collaborative response by the various agencies bridging city and county boundaries.

This outbreak had a significant impact on the resources of New York City, four counties, three states, and multiple federal agencies, yet it involved relatively few cases and deaths.[8] In the event of a bioterrorist attack with a rapidly increasing case count, decision making and response may need to be compressed to hours instead of days and weeks. This maximizes the risk of problems and errors.

The local public health departments know their communities and should work with their state health departments to develop or use already prepared fact sheets, problem alerts, training methods, communications systems, surveillance systems, plans, and protocols. They also should participate in periodic training exercises. At a minimum, regional and state partners must share plans when they are developed and constantly look to improve them.

Somewhat different grades of response are called for depending on whether a bioterrorist threat is used

Table 1

Public health planning requirements for a bioterrorism event

Health agencies	Components	Comments
Local	*Planning*	
	Emergency Management Plan	• Incorporate bioterrorism (BT) event response into existing emergency management plan
	Working relationships	• Review/develop protocols and working relationships with many agencies, including local government administrators in neighboring counties, offices of emergency management, local fire and police departments, local hospitals and providers, local FBI (office of first response), and local press, radio, and TV • Work with health providers on plans for mass medical care, including mass prophylaxis, mortuary care, and infection control; utilize existing documents such as the Association of Practitioners in Infection Control (APIC) BT readiness plan
	Interagency communication	• Improve links between health department, police, and FBI and plan together; the health department should notify the police and FBI of suspicious clusters of illness and the police and FBI should notify the health department of suspected BT activity
	Establish protocols	• Have *written* standards and protocols for response and consequence management
	Education/training	• Increase awareness of BT in medical community to improve rapid reporting of: – suspect cases potentially BT-related – unusual clusters of disease – unusual manifestations of disease, e.g., a flu-like illness with a widening mediastinum in a healthy adult = anthrax
	Surveillance	
	Reporters/information sources	• Surveillance might include: Emergency department reports for unusual patterns, hospital ICP and lab reports, electronic mortality reporting, medical examiner reports, geographic 911 analysis, poison control call, FBI, police, EMS activity, annual outbreaks, or unusual mortality patterns
	Influenza-like illness	• Improve surveillance for influenza-like illness, especially without URI symptoms because most BT agents present as flu-like illness • Sentinel networks are needed, monitor emergency departments, hospital admissions, employee health, schools, and EMS/911 calls
	Mortality reports	• Develop systems to more closely monitor unexplained deaths/illness possibly due to infectious causes (electronic death registry)
	Syndromic surveillance	• Establish surveillance criteria for emerging infections, looking for certain syndromes, e.g., pneumonia/fever with rash
	Resources	• All of the surveillance activity outlined may be limited by resources; planning includes maximizing resources to help accomplish the most important components of surveillance • New partners, new sources, new approaches need to be developed • Planning must be realistic

continues

Table 1

Continued

Health agencies	Components	Comments
State/major cities	*Planning*	
	Planning partners	• State departments of health should work closely with many agencies in the planning process including: – crisis and consequence management units; state police, FBI, EMS, State Emergency Management Office (SEMO) – local/regional health units/departments – other states/government entities
	Surveillance	• Items needed in plan: – surveillance systems for detecting BT or natural disease events, e.g., symptoms—cluster/syndromic surveillance techniques – protocols for large-scale surveillance and epidemiological investigations
	Laboratory support	• Develop state laboratory capacity to rapidly identify or rule out BT agents
	Communication	• Communication is critical between medical community and intelligence agencies and between government and the public
	Communication network	• Where possible, develop or expand on information infrastructure used by state and local health professionals to detect, respond to, and manage large-scale public health emergencies
	Alert distribution	• The systems should enable rapid dissemination of appropriate information to those that need to know • By design, it should link existing state, county, and hospital technology
	Local health/medical provider support	• Develop or adapt for distribution: – protocols on medical management and infection control of likely BT agents for distribution to providers – guidelines for mass medical care, including mass prophylaxis and mortuary care – identify facility needs: drugs, vaccines, equipment, staffing, etc. – outlines for handling events/threats/hoaxes – clinical diagnostic and treatment protocols – basic BT agent information for health care providers – laboratory, testing protocols – assorted planning documents, forms, and protocols (make available on communication network)
	Education/training	• Provide consultation/education • Develop laboratory criteria to educate clinical microbiologists when to report suspicious laboratory findings • Conduct periodic, multiagency training exercises, evaluating, and retraining

as a hoax, for extortion, or in the worst-case scenario as an unannounced large-scale event. National civil defense and emergency management planners have made it known in various ways that in terms of planning, federal responses will begin after the first 1,000 casualties, in general, and that support will take 12 to 36 hours to begin to arrive. Thus, planners should anticipate that communities/states are on their own for the first day or so.

The public health responses to a bioterrorism threat (surveillance, confirmation, communication) should be folded into current emergency management planning. The public health and medical response must include the items in Table 1.

REFERENCES

1. J. Reno, "The Threat of Chemical and Biological Weapons," Statement before the States Senate Committee on the Judiciary), Washington, DC, 22 April 1998.
2. Mary Woodard Lasker Charitable Trust. "Comment: Bioterrorism, FAST FACTS." http://laskercomment.com/comment/11/comm3.htm. Accessed August 4, 1999.
3. IQuest News. "News Release: Witnesses Endorse Nunn-Lugar-Domenici Program." http://web.iquest.net/lugar/rg1043298.html. Accessed April 8, 1999.
4. R.A. Clark, "Finding the Right Balance Against Bioterrorism." *Journal of Emerging Infectious Diseases* 5 (July/August 1999): 497–504.
5. J.E. McDade and D. Franz, "Bioterrorism as a Public Health Threat," *Journal of Emerging Infectious Diseases* (July/September 1998): 493–499.
6. T.J. Torok, et al., "A Large Community Outbreak of Salmonellosis Caused by Intentional Contamination of Restaurant Salad Bars," *JAMA* 278 (1997): 389–395.
7. J.M. Hughes, "The Emerging Threat of Bioterrorism," *Journal of Emerging Diseases* 5 (July/August 1999): 492–495.
8. A. Fine et al. "CDC Update: West Nile-Like Viral Encephalitis—New York, 1999," *Morbidity and Mortality Weekly Report* 48 (1999): 890–892, 944–955.

Commentary

The Role and Responsibility of the Media in the Event of a Bioterrorist Act

Hugh W. Wyatt

The role of the media will be critical if terrorists attack the civilian population of the United States with germ or chemical warfare. Although the motivation of the group may vary, one aim of the bioterrorists will be to create panic at all levels of society. The media's response must be responsible reporting.

THE ROLE OF THE news media will be critical if terrorists attack the civilian population of the United States with germ or chemical warfare. Although the motivation of the group may vary, one aim of the bioterrorists will be to create panic at all levels of society. The media's response must be responsible reporting. Sensational, irresponsible coverage of a massive anthrax outbreak, for example, would play into the hands of the bioterrorists and lead to chaos in the streets of both big cities and small communities. There are times when all of us in the media must defer to responsible government institutions, just as automobile drivers defer to a police officer who is directing traffic. If recent events are an example (see Cole's article in this issue), the media must not create controversy and sensationalism in order to improve ratings.

In the event of an anthrax scare, local radio and TV stations may be tempted to put an "expert" on the air with advice on what to do. Such "experts" are likely to be drawn from the private sector, but even the best infectious disease specialists in our hospitals lack experience, training, and knowledge about a disease like anthrax. Responding to media questions by translating their expertise on common communicable diseases can result in inappropriate guidance. If these specialists disagree with one another, or with the official government announcements, a much more serious consequence results—cognitive dissonance. The public will become confused, terrified, and distrustful; it may conclude that no one knows

Hugh W. Wyatt *is Editor and Publisher of the* Medical Herald *in New York, New York.*

how to deal with the crisis. Official local, state, and federal government warnings and requests may not be heeded.

Those who have studied bioterrorism—such as D.A. Henderson, MD, Director of the Johns Hopkins Center for Civilian Bio-Defense Studies—believe that smallpox and anthrax are the two weapons of greatest concern. Anthrax spores, drifting silently across a city, would be invisible, odorless, tasteless, and lethal to 80 percent of those exposed to them. Bioterrorists could also release germs that cause plague, another bacterial disease that can also be spread in the air through a spray. Unlike anthrax (or tularemia), primary victims of pneumonic plague are infectious to others, including family, friends, and primary health care providers. Tularemia (rabbit fever) is a cousin of plague and although airborne, it can contaminate food and water supplies. The same is true of botulinum toxin, which, under proper circumstances, can be airborne, foodborne, and waterborne. Henderson stated:

> Recent events in Iraq, Japan and Russia cast an ominous shadow over the whole world. Iraq has admitted to having weapons that contain anthrax and botulism. The cult that released nerve gas in the Tokyo subway in 1995 also had (or has) an arsenal of biological weapons. Military scientists in the former Soviet Union are known to have worked long and hard on biological weapons, including smallpox, Ebola, Marburg and hemorrhagic fever viruses.[1(p.489)]

National policy makers and academics once treated bioterrorism as nothing more than a theoretical possibility. This is no longer the case. It is time to take the threat of bioterrorism seriously and to admit that the U.S. is nowhere near to being adequately prepared to defend itself and its communities from either a military enemy or a determined madman.

In the event of an outbreak of one or more epidemics of disease caused by terrorists, it will be the responsibility of the media to focus on the people with the real answers. They include the Centers for Disease Control and Prevention (CDC) in Atlanta, the U.S. Surgeon General, the Public Health Service, and other federal, state, and local agencies. Equally important to this process is the local media—those newspapers, radio stations, and television stations with loyal followings. Newspaper editors, columnists, radio talk show personalities, and television reporters who are known and respected will be followed carefully. These individuals should reinforce the messages delivered by the anonymous names and faces of government agencies. To not do so—unless there are clear indications of error—would be a disservice to the public.

An example of irresponsible reporting was the coverage of an outbreak of legionnaires' disease in Philadelphia in the summer of 1976. There were 182 cases of the disease among people attending an American Legion convention.[2] When the disease was recognized, panic fed by media reports spread not only in the streets of Philadelphia but throughout Pennsylvania and the nation. Months later, it was established that the disease could not be spread from one individual to another. If bioterrorists strike the United States, federal and state governments have a number of Internet sites that will be available to assist the public, the media, and others regarding what to do. New York City is considered the most likely target for an initial terrorist attack. The Mayor's Office of Emergency Management has established an emergency command post on the 23rd floor of a building adjacent to the World Trade Center. Responses to various situations were organized at the Mayor's Office of Emergency Management, including a hurricane threat, the West Nile Virus outbreak, a blackout, building collapses, and major breaks in sewer lines leading to flooding. Jerome M. Hauer, the former leader of the Mayor's Office of Emergency Management, and other experienced individuals in similar positions are exactly the kind of people the media should keep closely in touch with to get the latest and most accurate information about an attack. That will be responsible reporting.

I believe the media also would do well to voluntarily establish guidelines in advance on how to cover bioterrorism outbreaks. Executives from the top newspapers and television and radio networks should establish these guidelines in cooperation with responsible government officials. The same process then should be followed by local newspapers, radio stations, and local television stations. Most county, city, and state health agencies, as well as emergency medical services, should be willing to discuss their scenarios to deal with a bioterrorism attack. If they cannot or will not, they are appropriate targets for media criticism before such an event were to happen.

In addition to New York City, Washington, DC, is considered a likely target for terrorists because of the embassies, monuments, and federal agencies there. In response to threats of chemical, biological, or nuclear terrorism, the Federal Bureau of Investigation's Washington field office has set up a counter-terrorist squad called the National Capital Domestic Response Squad. The squad includes a 50-member special weapons and tactics team, a bomb squad, a 20-member hazardous materials team, and a medical unit. The head of the squad, James Rice, says the group is working with law enforcement and security officials drawn from 12 local and federal agencies. Other cities and counties should seek their counterpart to Rice ahead of time as a source of accurate and reliable information.

The media will have a particular responsibility to city dwellers in such cities as New York and Washington who are not affluent and will not be able to escape to faraway retreats in the case of an emergency. These people, including minority residents of inner-city communities, will be dependent on the accuracy of reports in newspapers, the Internet, radio, and TV. Unlike commuters or the more mobile, affluent classes, they won't have the ability to escape very far. If there is irresponsible reporting, this vulnerable group will be terrified and may panic. This could lead to a scenario in which otherwise permanent city residents flee to the suburbs with little resources. They may arrive in suburbs and exurbs hungry, homeless, and desperate. Locals would be terrified of contagion; law enforcement agencies would be overwhelmed. Some citizens might form vigilante groups, further testing finite law enforcement agencies. Once again, this would play into the hands of the bioterrorists because their aim would be to paralyze the United States. The media also would do well to study the reports of such institutions as the Johns Hopkins Center for Civilian Bio-Defense Studies (the Center) in Baltimore, headed by D.A. Henderson. These reports provide accurate previews of what to expect if the worst happens. In a report on smallpox, for example, the Center said this disease represents one of the most serious threats to the civilian population because of its high fatality rates and its transmissibility.[3]

Over the centuries, naturally occurring smallpox—with its fatality rate of 30 percent or more and its ability to spread in any climate and season—has been feared universally as the most devastating of all the infectious diseases. Smallpox was worldwide in scope before vaccination was practiced. In 1980, the World Health Assembly announced that smallpox had been eradicated. It recommended that all countries cease vaccination. But in the same year, the Soviet government embarked on an ambitious program to grow smallpox virus in large quantities and adapt it for use in bombs and intercontinental ballistic missiles.

Russia still possesses an industrial facility that is capable of producing smallpox virus. An aerosol release of smallpox virus could infect thousands of people. There would be an interval of close to two weeks before the disease was diagnosed. This is because there is an average incubation period of 12 to 14 days. After the incubation period, a patient experiences high fever, malaise, and prostration with headache and backache. Severe abdominal pain and delirium are sometimes present. A smallpox outbreak poses difficult problems because of the ability of the virus to continue to spread throughout the population unless checked by vaccination and/or isolation of patients and their close contacts.

Approximately 140,000 vials of vaccine are in storage at the CDC, each with doses for 50 to 60 people. An additional 50 million to 100 million doses are estimated to exist worldwide. This stock cannot be replenished immediately because all vaccine production facilities were dismantled after 1980. There are no proven antiviral agents effective in treating smallpox.

All major scourges have had a profound impact on human history. The first great plague pandemic began in Egypt in 541 and swept over the world in four years, killing an estimated 50 to 60 percent of the known world's population.[4] A second plague pandemic began in 1346 and killed one third of the population of Europe.[4] Advances in living conditions, public health, and antibiotic therapy make it unlikely that there will ever be another natural plague pandemic, but these lessons from history underscore an innate fear the public shares about contagious diseases.

There is a thin veneer of civilization between the Europe of 800 years ago and today. Scratch the surface and the fatuity placed in modern-day medicine may disappear. Fear, panic, and perhaps chaos may follow after an outbreak of plague occurs and the government and public infrastructures collapse. Witness a recent example: plague caused widespread panic after the discovery of even a small number of cases. An estimated 500,000 persons fled the city of Surat, India, in 1994 in fear of a plague epidemic. In the 1950s and 1960s, Soviet biological programs developed techniques to aerosolize plague particles, a technique that leads to pneumonic plague, an otherwise uncommon but highly lethal form of the disease.[5] More than 10 institutes and thousands of scientists were reported to have worked with plague in the former Soviet Union. The size of a pneumonic plague epidemic after an aerosol attack would depend on a number of factors including the amount of agent used, the meteorological conditions, and the method of aerosolization and dissemination. There are no effective environmental warning systems to detect an aerosol cloud of plague bacilli and there are no widely available rapid diagnostic tests. The mortality of untreated pneumonic plague cases approaches 100 percent.

Anthrax infection is a disease acquired following contact with infected animals or contaminated animal products. In the second half of the 20th century, anthrax was developed as part of a larger biological weapons program in several countries, including the former Soviet Union. Given appropriate weather and wind conditions, 50 kilograms of anthrax released from an airplane could create a lethal cloud of anthrax spores that would extend more than 20 kilometers downwind. The aerosol cloud would be colorless, odorless, and invisible. The spores are so small that people indoors would receive the same amount of exposure as people on the street. There are no atmospheric warning systems to detect an aerosol cloud of anthrax spores.

An analysis by the Congressional Office of Technology Assessment estimated that 130,000 to three million deaths could occur following the release of 100 kilograms of aerosolized anthrax over Washington, DC, making the attack as lethal as a hydrogen bomb. The largest experience with inhalation anthrax occurred after the accidental release of aerosolized anthrax spores in 1979 at a military biology facility in Sverdlovsk, Russia. Seventy-nine cases of inhalation anthrax were reported, of which 68 were fatal.[6] The United States has developed an anthrax vaccine for use by military personnel, but there is no vaccine available for civilian use.

■ ■ ■

The threat of bioterrorism is real. It cannot be ignored by the media. In wartime, the media has engaged in voluntary self-policing. During World War II, no newspaper or broadcast organization would have carried a report giving aid or comfort to the Germans or Japanese. Indeed, the Japanese sent scores of balloons from the main island of Japan across the Pacific, riding the jet stream thousands of miles and landing in California, Washington, and as far east as Ann Arbor, Michigan. The balloons carried incendiaries that caused fires throughout the western states. However, Washington censored all reports of fires. The Japanese concluded that the balloons fell into the Pacific Ocean and decided not to launch other balloons carrying plague, anthrax, and other deadly infectious agents. This example of censorship may have been extreme; however, it was successful. Less stringent self-censorship might be exercised by today's media in order to prevent a bioterrorist group to claim success. The policy of self-policing and accurate, responsible reporting must be followed in the event of a bioterrorist attack and the time to prepare for such reporting is now.

REFERENCES

1. D.A. Henderson, "Bioterrorism as a Public Health Threat," *Emerging Infectious Diseases* 4, no. 3 (July/September 1998): 488–492.
2. D.W. Fraser, et al., "Legionnaires' Disease: Descriptions of An Epidemic of Pneumonia," *New England Journal of Medicine* 297, no. 22 (1977): 1189–1197.
3. D.A. Henderson, "Smallpox: Clinical and Epidemiologic Features," *Emerging Infectious Diseases* 5, no. 4 (July/August 1999): 537–539.
4. S. Tenner and A. Schamess, "Pandemic, Medicine, and Public Health: Yersinia Pestis and Fourteenth Century European Culture," *Pharos Fall* 56, no. 4 (1993): 6–10.
5. J. Stern, "The Prospect of Domestic Bioterrorism," *Emerg Infectious Disease* 5, no. 4 (July/August 1994): 517–522.
6. M. Meselson et al., "The Sverdlovsk Anthrax Outbreak of 1979," *Science* 266, no. 5188 (18 November 1994): 1202–1208.

Internet Resources Related to Biological and Chemical Terrorism

THE UBIQUITY OF the Internet provides public health specialists access to an abundance of information on all topics, including appropriate responses to terrorist events. The Internet addresses provided below represent a cross-section of the many sites devoted to biological and chemical terrorism. Due to the dynamic nature of the World Wide Web, the contents of some sites and their addresses may change. An attempt was made to provide information on more established sites that will remain in existence for years to come.

These sites are divided into media, governmental, and nongovernmental. Among the medical media sites, access to some locations is free (such as http://www.medscape.com), while other addresses currently require a subscription to the accompanying paper-based publication (such as http://www.thelancet.com and http://www.nejm.org). Not included in the media resources list are lay media news sites, which are abundant on the web (including the *New York Times*, the *Washington Post*, CNN, MSNBC, and so forth). These sites generally provide news articles of threats, preparatory efforts, opinions, and editorials related to biological and chemical terrorism. Most lay media sites have a search engine that will locate recent articles related to any subject of interest.

The governmental and military sites, all of which are specific to the United States, provide substantive information, reports, and guidelines. The *Morbidity and Mortality Weekly Report* link provides the publication, "Bioterrorism: Alleging Use of Anthrax and Interim Guidelines for Management—United States, 1998." Readers are encouraged to use the search function on the governmental sites, particularly at the site administered by the Centers for Disease Control and Prevention, to locate newly published guidelines and reports. The final link in this section is to PubMed, the National Library of Medicine's comprehensive database of peer-reviewed publications.

Nongovernment sites include both for-profit organizations related to preparedness (such as http://www.terrorism.com and http://www.emergency.com) as well as not-for-profit organizations and foundations (including the Federation of American Scientists, the Henry L. Stimson Center, the Mary Woodard Lasker Charitable Trust, and others). Program for Monitoring Emerging Diseases is a unique Internet-based global surveillance system for the early detection of emerging infectious diseases and indeed may yield the first indication of an incident of chemical or biological terrorism.

The Web, with its abundance of information, is a tool that should be employed, albeit with prudent evaluation, by all public health professionals. Search engines such as http://www.hotbot.com, http://www.google.com, and http://www.dogpile.com assist in the location of information on a variety of issues relevant to public health professionals. As with all information available on the Internet, it is critical to evaluate the quality of the content of each site.

Medical and Scientific Media Sites

1. http://jama.ama-assn.org/
2. http://www.nejm.org/
3. http://www.thelancet.com/
4. http://www.bmj.com/
5. http://www.newscientist.com/
6. http://www.medscape.com
7. http://www.sciam.com/1296issue/1296cole.html

Government Sites

1. http://www.cdc.gov/ncidod/eid/
2. http://www.cdc.gov/epo/mmwr/preview/mmwrhtml/00056353.htm
3. http://www.cdc.gov/phtn/bioterrorism/factsheet.htm
4. http://www.cdc.gov/ncidod/dbmd/diseaseinfo/default.htm
5. http://www.nih.gov/news/NIH-Record/04_20_99/story01.htm
6. http://dp.sbccom.army.mil/au.html
7. http://www.usamriid.army.mil/
8. http://www.fema.gov/rris/
9. http://www.ncbi.nlm.nih.gov/entrez/query.fcgi?db=PubMed

Nongovernment Sites

1. http://www.fas.org/bwc/
2. http://osi.oracle.com:8080/promed/promed.home
3. http://www.hopkins-biodefense.org/
4. http://www.laskerfoundation.org/fundingfirst/comment/11/index.html
5. http://www.stimson.org/cwc/index.html
6. http://www.potomacinstitute.com/projects/cbt/cbt.htm
7. http://www.terrorism.com/
8. http://www.emergency.com

Public Health Grand Rounds Addresses Bioterrorism Preparedness

William L. Roper and Donna E. Davis

THE SCHOOL OF Public Health at The University of North Carolina at Chapel Hill (UNC–SPH) has collaborated with the Centers for Disease Control and Prevention (CDC) to launch Public Health Grand Rounds, a series of programs on contemporary public health issues aimed at educating health leaders and practitioners. The first edition was a satellite broadcast and Web cast titled "Bioterrorism: Implications for Public Health," which aired June 11, 1999. It brought together an estimated 4,200 public health and safety professionals at 389 sites from all 50 states and Canada. Public Health Grand Rounds is a product of a multiagency partnership that includes CDC's Public Health Training Network, the Association of Schools of Public Health, the National Association of County and City Health Officials (NACCHO), and the Association of State and Territorial Health Officials (ASTHO).

Public Health Grand Rounds is moderated by William L. Roper, MD, MPH, Dean of UNC–SPH, and the case presenter is Hugh H. Tilson, MD, DrPH, Clinical Professor of Epidemiology and Health Policy at UNC–SPH. Jeffrey P. Koplan, MD, MPH, Director of the CDC, co-moderated the inaugural broadcast. The content expert changes with each program. With "Bioterrorism: Implications for Public Health," it was Scott R. Lillibridge, MD, Director of the Office of Bioterrorism Preparedness and Response at the CDC.

Through in-depth analysis of real world health issues by experts in the science and practice of public health, Public Health Grand Rounds provides a forum through which health professionals and others can develop timely, reasoned, and productive responses to public health issues of regional and national significance. The series' telecommunications network creates a system for disseminating information relevant to the planning of prevention and intervention strategies for emergent public health issues.

The grand rounds model has long been a successful training tool used to teach physicians. In medical grand rounds, various medical specialists present their perspectives on the etiology, diagnosis, prognosis, and treatment plan for a patient's presenting problem to an audience of students, practicing physicians, and other medical professionals. Case histories are used to illustrate the clinical presentation of diseases, to provide a context in which participants can review basic information, and to focus discussion on several possible ways to frame and address the problem.[1]

In Public Health Grand Rounds, the "patient" is defined as the community and the "presenting problem" is defined as a public health issue currently challenging the community and requiring its informed response. As in medical grand rounds, a panel of expert "specialists" is assembled to provide the most current information and data related to the case and to assess the problem from the specialists' professional perspective, knowledge, and experience. The specialists and the audience in the Public Health Grand Rounds model are more professionally heterogeneous than in the medical grand rounds model, reflecting the greater complexity of the patient and the community.

William L. Roper, MD, MPH, *is Dean of the School of Public Health, University of North Carolina at Chapel Hill, Chapel Hill, North Carolina.*

Donna E. Davis, MPH, *is Project Director, Public Health Grand Rounds, the North Carolina Institute for Public Health, the University of North Carolina at Chapel Hill.*

Indianapolis was the community featured in the inaugural broadcast. On October 30, 1998, this city faced a bioterrorist threat involving a powdery substance purported to be anthrax. Fortunately, this was discovered to be a hoax.[2] Community leaders spoke with Tilson about how a strong public health infrastructure contributed to their quick response. They were very candid about their strengths and weaknesses as well as the lessons they learned. The moderators led a discussion with the national audience on important elements and implications of the public health's role in bioterrorism response. An archived version of this program can be found at http://www.publichealthgrandrounds.unc.edu.

Infrastructure is a common theme with all of the Grand Rounds programs. An underlying goal is to improve local, state, and federal public health infrastructure by featuring exemplary cases where public health challenges have been overcome by agencies working together. Establishing good working relationships before the occurrence of a bioterrorism incident is the key to protecting the health of a community in the wake of such a disaster. These relationships will also help the community address other contemporary public health challenges. Subsequent grand rounds programs on breast cancer screening and disaster preparedness also emphasized the importance of a strong public health infrastructure.

Another common theme of the Public Health Grand Rounds series is technology. As mentioned earlier, the series uses satellite and Web cast technology to deliver programs to all 50 states and Canada. This program was the first of its kind to require registration through the Internet. Program materials, notes, resources, and a printable brochure also were made available at the program Web site (http://www.publichealthgrandrounds.unc.edu). A total of 1,685 participants completed an on-line registration for "Bioterrorism: Implications for Public Health." These registrations comprised a diverse audience whose professions varied from paramedic to local health director. Nearly 400 nurses, 166 environmental health specialists, 153 laboratorians, and 140 physicians registered to attend. More than 42 percent of those registered were affiliated with a local health department, 13 percent were from clinical settings, and 7 percent represented educational and research organizations. Without the technology of the Internet, this information would have been gathered at great expense, both in time and resources.

With Internet technology, Public Health Grand Rounds is paving the way for the public health work force to be trained and educated in the 21st century. One of the greatest accomplishments of this series is that it was shared with public health professionals from across the nation without the expense and inconvenience of travel. Eighty-six percent of the evaluations indicated that fewer than 20 miles were traveled to attend. Nearly 50 participants watched the program live from their desktops through a Web cast supported by streaming video.

The challenge of preparing communities for possible bioterrorism incidents is an awesome task. It will require the coordinated efforts of those already engaged in training the public health work force, for example, schools of public health, federal agencies such as the CDC and the Health Resources and Services Administration, and national organizations such as ASTHO and NACCHO. Use of satellite broadcast and Web cast technology will carry the message of preparedness to those who would otherwise be out of reach. The convenience and easy access of the Internet will make information readily available to public health leaders and practitioners seeking to educate themselves on this latest public health challenge. For more information on the Public Health Grand Rounds series, please contact project director Donna E. Davis, MPH, at donna_davis@unc.edu or 919-966-9134.

REFERENCES

1. D. Schon, *Educating the Reflective Practitioner*. San Francisco: Jossey-Bass, 1987.
2. "Bioterrorism Alleging Use of Anthrax and Interim Guidelines for Management—United States, 1998," *Morbidity and Mortality Weekly Report* 48, no. 4 (February 5, 1999 / 48(04): 69–74.

Prioritization Methods for HIV Community Planning

Ana P. Johnson-Masotti, Steven D. Pinkerton, and David R. Holtgrave

Since 1994, community planning groups (CPGs) have played an important role in shaping local HIV prevention efforts. The community planning process requires CPGs to prioritize HIV prevention interventions and unmet needs among at-risk populations. This article describes and compares four prioritization methods: (1) the ranking method, (2) Holtgrave's method, (3) Kaplan's method, and (4) a novel utility-based prioritization method. These methods are compared in terms of effectiveness, efficiency, equity, and political feasibility. The methods described here are meant to assist CPGs in the difficult prioritization task by helping CPG members organize their thoughts in the prioritization process.

Introduction

In 1993, the Centers for Disease Control and Prevention (CDC) issued a program guidance to its 65 health department grantees who received federal human immunodeficiency virus (HIV) prevention funds, formally establishing local HIV prevention "community planning groups" (CPGs).[1] CPGs are composed of members of HIV-infected and affected communities, behavioral scientists, epidemiologists and other technical experts, representatives from the state or local health department, and staff from nongovernment organizations and departments of health and education as well as substance abuse prevention. The main charge of CPGs is to identify unmet HIV prevention needs, based on sound epidemiological evidence, and to identify and prioritize HIV prevention intervention that could be undertaken to address these unmet needs.[2,3]

This study was supported in part by Center Grant P30–MH52776 from the National Institute of Mental Health and through the second author's Interagency Personnel Agreement with the Centers for Disease Control and Prevention.

Ana P. Johnson-Masotti, PhD, *is Assistant Professor at the Center for AIDS Intervention Research, Department of Psychiatry and Behavioral Medicine, Medical College of Wisconsin in Milwaukee.*

Steven D. Pinkerton, PhD, *is Director of the Cost-Effective Studies Core at the Center for AIDS Intervention Research, Department of Psychiatry and Behavioral Medicine, Medical College of Wisconsin in Milwaukee.*

David R. Holtgrave, PhD, *is the Director of the Division of HIV/AIDS Prevention—Intervention Research and Support, National Center for HIV, STD, and TB Prevention, Centers for Disease Control and Prevention in Atlanta, Georgia.*

The final "product" of the community planning process for a given year is a prioritization plan that is based on identified needs and prevention programs to address those needs. The plan is delivered to state or local health department officials, who then develop a request for CDC funding based on the plan. Finally, the funding request is sent to the CDC, where allocation of resources for the following fiscal year is determined based on the health department's request, national prevention goals, and other considerations.[2–4]

The CDC's guidance on community planning lists seven factors that CPGs should explicitly consider when prioritizing interventions:[1,4]

1. documented HIV prevention needs based on current and projected impact of HIV/acquired immune deficiency syndrome (AIDS) in defined populations
2. outcome effectiveness of proposed strategies and interventions (either demonstrated or probable)
3. cost-effectiveness of proposed strategies and interventions (either demonstrated or probable)
4. sound scientific theory (e.g., behavior change, social change, and social marketing theories)
5. values, norms, and consumer preferences of the communities for which the services are intended
6. availability of other government and nongovernment resources (including the private sector) for HIV prevention
7. other factors that may be of local significance

Beyond these explicit considerations, CPGs have considerable freedom in how they go about prioritizing interventions. Some CPGs use numerical weighting or "group consensus" methods to rank priority programs.[5] Others have adopted one or more of the priority setting tools described in the Academy for Educational Development (AED)/CDC publication, *"Handbook for HIV Prevention Community Planning,"*[6] which is available through the CDC's National Technical Assistance Network. The AED/CDC document describes several prioritization methods including the nominal group method, in which a facilitator poses thought-provoking questions to CPG members to help them think through the decision making process; the rating/ranking method (described below) wherein CPG members rate or rank interventions and populations in need of HIV prevention based on preselected criteria; and the Delphi method, in which priorities are determined through an iterative process of expert opinion solicitation and reconciliation.[6–8] More complex prioritization models have also been described in the scientific literature, notably by Holtgrave[4] and Kaplan.[9]

Prioritization is an inherently difficult task that is complicated by a number of factors, including the wide range of diverse populations and perspectives represented by CPG members; the need to synthesize disparate types of information such as behavioral risk profiles, data on the local epidemiology of HIV, and information on the effectiveness and cost-effectiveness of various HIV prevention interventions; and difficulties in obtaining the data needed to implement the prioritization models described above.[7] The last problem appears to be especially widespread.[10] Both Holtgrave's and Kaplan's prioritization models, and to a lesser extent the AED/CDC methods, require very specific information on the impact of candidate interventions, which in turn is a complex function of intervention effectiveness, local epidemiology, and existing population risk levels. Often, the only source of such data is expert opinion. Moreover, it is difficult to integrate these "objective" data with anecdotal data, values, norms, opinions, and local politics, all of which are important concerns to CPG members.[11]

In this article, we review four different methods for prioritizing HIV interventions and unmet needs: the ranking method, two more complex techniques suggested by Holtgrave and Kaplan, and a novel utility-based prioritization method for use by CPGs. This method permits CPG members to assign subjectively determined weights to different data-related criteria and value-related criteria and thereby incorporate into the decision-making process judgments about the quality or importance of the data as well as the data themselves. After reviewing/introducing the four methods, we discuss their advantages and disadvantages and their role in the decision-making process.

Priority Setting Models

Formal decision-making models can be used to help CPGs with the difficult task of prioritizing HIV prevention needs and interventions to serve those needs. Below, we describe four of the methods available to CPGs: (1) the ranking method, (2) Holtgrave's priority setting model, (3) Kaplan's resource allocation model, and (4) the utility-based prioritization method.

The ranking technique

The ranking technique is a prioritization method in which CPG members rank interventions or populations according to preselected criteria.[6,7] It has been offered to local health departments in the United States and in developing countries to aid their organizational capacity, strengthen their leadership role in the community, and design public health programs.[12–14] More recently, it has been used to rank Oregon's Medicaid lists;[15] to rank views on priorities for health services;[16] to identify which pesticides would be targeted for a brain cancer case-control study;[17] and to prioritize topics for future research in emergency medical services for children.[18] Its effectiveness has been assessed in the field of occupational medicine; in identifying areas of priority in occupational health;[19] in the pharmaceutical industry;[20] in priority setting at the District Health Authority level in Britain;[21] and in comparison with the contingent valuation ranking method.[22]

For the ranking method, the criteria could include any of a number of dimensions such as intervention effectiveness (actual or estimated), expected sustainability of the intervention, or the prevalence of HIV infection or need for prevention efforts in a particular population. Competing interventions (or population groups) are ranked on each of the criteria and then the rankings are combined into overall scores for the different interventions. The intervention (or population) that receives the highest priority is the one with the lowest overall score. Because it requires CPG members to explicitly compare each intervention or population with every other one, this method works best when the number of interventions or populations is small.[7]

When prioritizing interventions using the ranking method, the first step is to develop the list of criteria. This can be done through a group consensus method in which CPG members suggest possible criteria until an exhaustive list has been compiled. This list can be paired down by voting on whether each of the listed criteria should be retained or removed from the list. The next step is for each CPG member to assign a ranking to each intervention based on these criteria. Finally, the overall score for each intervention is calculated by summing up the rankings it received on the criteria. For example, suppose that three interventions (A_1, A_2, and A_3) are ranked on three criteria (effectiveness, sustainability, and cost) as follows: effectiveness (#1 rank = A_1; #2 rank = A_2; #3 rank = A_3); sustainability (#1 rank = A_1; #2 rank = A_3; #3 rank = A_2); and cost (#1 rank = A_3; #2 rank = A_2; #3 rank = A_1). By assigning one point for each #1 ranking that an intervention receives, two points for each #2 ranking, and three points for each #3 ranking, the overall scores for interventions A_1, A_2, and A_3 are 5 (1+1+3), 7 (2+3+2), and 6 (3+2+1), respectively.

So far, we have discussed a single CPG member. Now imagine that every CPG member has followed this procedure individually to come up with his or her own set of overall scores. For instance, if there are five CPG members, perhaps intervention A_1 received scores of 5, 5, 6, 4, and 5; intervention A_2 received scores of 7, 6, 4, 8, and 7; and intervention A_3 received scores of 6, 7, 8, 6, and 6. The corresponding total scores are 25, 32, and 33. Hence, based on this exercise, intervention A_1 would receive the highest priority (because it has the lowest total score), followed by intervention A_2, and then intervention A_3. Note that averaging these rankings is technically not appropriate (although very often conducted). The rating method has been used in Florida, for example.[23]

Holtgrave's priority setting method

Holtgrave[4] developed a simple method for prioritizing HIV prevention programs to address unmet needs in the community. This model is based on the multiattribute utility theory (MAUT) and has been developed to assist local decision makers in developing countries.[24] General software is available for general MAUT application.[25] Multiattribute utility techniques have been used more recently for obtaining patient values on periodontal health;[26] in the decision of nursing students in Taiwan to be vaccinated against hepatitis B infection;[27] in identifying areas of family life most affected by childhood atopic dermatitis;[28] for assessing patient perceptions on the impact of menorrhagia on their health;[29] and in the Alzheimer's framework.[30] The effectiveness of the multiattribute utility decision framework was assessed in groups for personnel selection problems differing in complexity;[31] among university students; and among Alzheimer patients.[30]

There are five steps in Holtgrave's algorithm:

1. Members of the CPG identify unmet HIV prevention needs in the relevant jurisdiction and then rank these needs according to the estimated number of HIV infections that would occur if a prevention program were not offered to meet these needs.
2. For each unmet need, the CPG generates a comprehensive list of appropriate prevention interventions to meet those unmet needs.
3. Potential interventions then must pass a three-pronged test: Is it legal? Is it accessible to the target community? Is it acceptable to that community? If the answer (determined by consensus) to any one question is "no," then the intervention is eliminated from the list of candidate interventions.
4. Each of the remaining interventions is awarded between zero to three points based on whether the intervention is believed or known to be effective, cost-effective, and based on behavioral science and social science theory. An intervention receives 1 point for each affirmative response to these three criteria (if information is lacking on one of these criteria, then the intervention can be awarded half a point). Thus, each prevention intervention has a score ranging from 0 to 3. (This scoring scheme can be altered to permit CPG members to assign more importance to one criterion or another. This could be accomplished, for example, by assigning up to two points to effective interventions so that total scores would range from 0 to 4, with effectiveness receiving twice the weight of either cost-effectiveness or grounding in the behavioral and social sciences.) An ineffective intervention is not likely to be selected because its effectiveness and cost-effectiveness scores would be zero.
5. Finally, the interventions for a particular unmet need are ranked according to their scores on the three criteria. Prevention interventions that meet all three criteria or the largest number of criteria (i.e., have the highest score) are preferred.

Overall, the highest priority intervention is the one that received the highest score (step #5) of those interventions that address the most important unmet need (step #1). The next highest priority is the top-scoring intervention that addresses the second most important need, and so forth. When an intervention has been selected for every unmet need, the second-highest ranking intervention for the most important unmet need would be selected, and so forth. This procedure is illustrated in Figure 1.

Next, we propose a novel extension of Holtgrave's method that can be used when quantitative estimates of the number of infections that could be prevented by the different interventions are available. This extension has five steps:

1. Identify all unmet HIV prevention needs in the relevant jurisdiction, but do not rank them yet.
2. For each unmet need, generate a comprehensive list of appropriate prevention interventions to meet those unmet needs.
3. Potential interventions must pass a five-pronged test: Is it legal? Is it accessible to the target community? Is it acceptable to that community? Is it effective? Is it cost-effective? A "no" response to any one of these questions eliminates the intervention from further consideration.
4. For each unmet need, rank the candidate interventions according to the number of infections they would prevent if implemented in the target community.
5. Prioritize the interventions across unmet need categories by first selecting the intervention that would prevent the most infections if implemented in its associated target community. Then reassess the unmet need for this community, taking into account the impact of the intervention. For example, if the original needs assessment indicated that there would be five infections in the target community if no interventions were implemented and the most effective intervention would avert three of these, then the residual unmet need is two potential infections. (If there is no residual need, then the community is excluded from further consideration.) The second highest priority intervention is the one that prevents the most interventions given that the highest priority intervention has been implemented already. This process, which is illustrated in Figure 2, continues until there are no more unmet needs in any community.

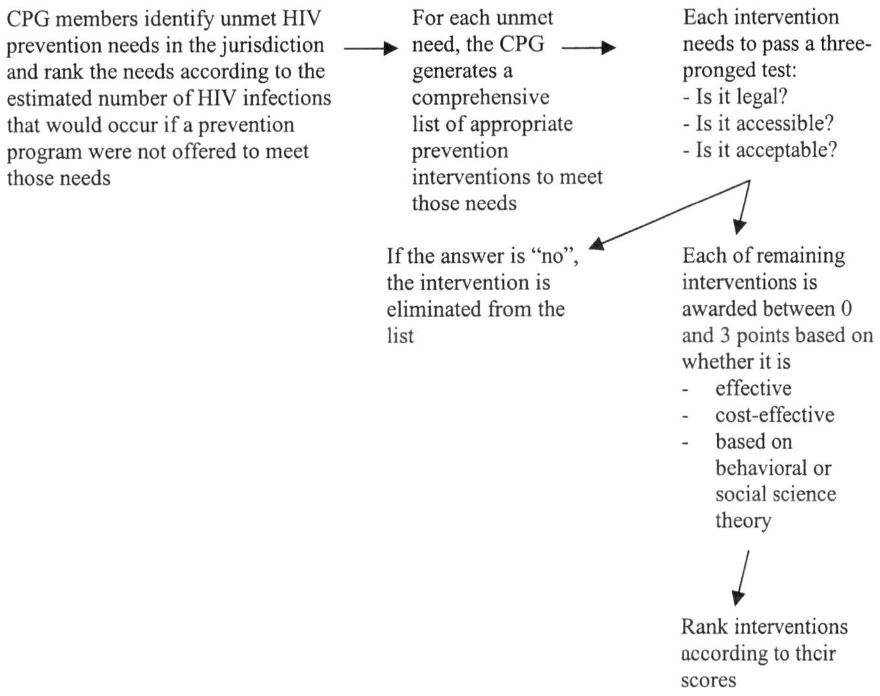

Figure 1. An algorithm illustrating Holtgrave's model

Importantly, the extension outlined above requires numerical estimates of unmet needs in target communities (i.e., the number of potential infections that would occur if no interventions were implemented) and the effectiveness of various interventions in meeting these needs (i.e., the number of infections that would be averted by the intervention). In contrast, the basic Holtgrave model requires only that unmet needs be ranked, therefore, relative rather than absolute estimates are all that are required. Thus, this extension has substantially greater data requirements than the original model.

Kaplan's resource allocation model

The goal of Kaplan's resource allocation model is to determine how HIV prevention funds should be allocated ideally to achieve the lowest levels of HIV infection in the target community.[9] It is derived from the field of economics in dividing budgets to achieve an objective.[32] More recently, the resource allocation method has been used as a guide for planning community-oriented health care;[33] in the field of substance abuse prevention;[34] and to enhance the productivity of academic physicians.[35] It has been assessed in the field of substance abuse prevention.[36]

Kaplan models the relationship between limited funds or resources and the number of HIV infections prevented as an economist would model the relationship between economic input and output (i.e., as a "production function"). The question is how many infections can be prevented by investing a given amount of money in a particular set of one or more HIV prevention interventions. This method tackles the implied resource allocation problem of specific allocations such as splitting the budget in proportion to HIV incidence, for example. It makes the budget allocation process explicit.[37] The input to the model is the monetary spending on HIV interventions, and the output is the resulting change in the expected number of HIV infections. It should be noted that at the outset, CPGs do not directly allocate funds—this is the responsibility of the health department. However, some CPGs do make allocation recommendations to their health departments.[2–4]

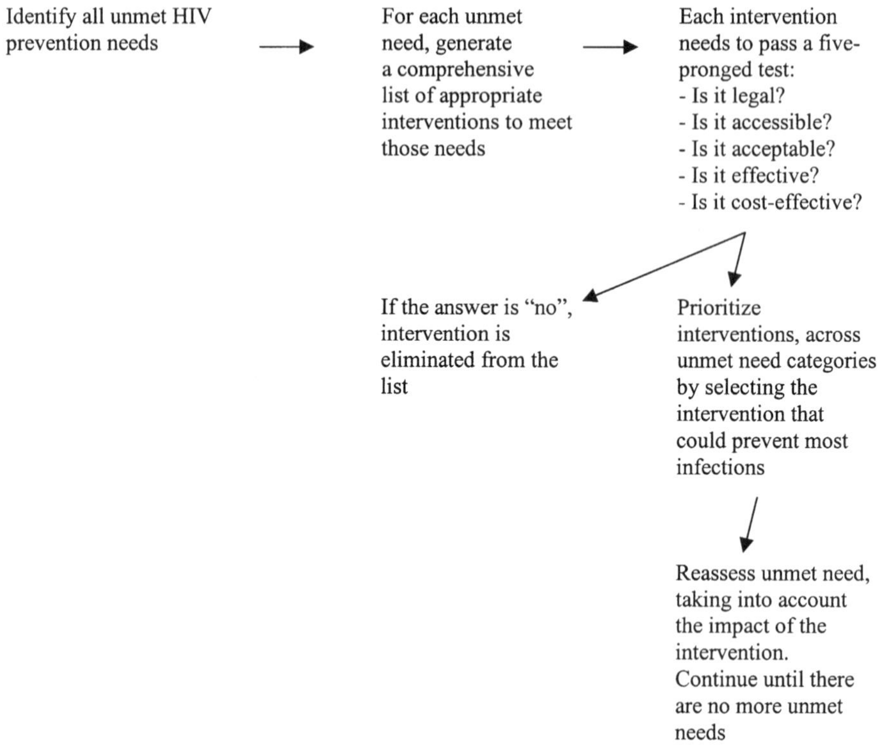

Figure 2. An algorithm illustrating a novel extension of Holtgrave's method

The main outcome measure, the change in the number of infections, $\Delta I(x)$, equals the number of new infections that would result during a specified length of time (one year, for example) if no money were invested in a particular HIV prevention intervention, $I(0)$, minus the number of new infections, $I(x)$, that would result if the intervention were implemented at a specified funding level (x) (in dollars). Symbolically, $\Delta I(x) = I(0) - I(x)$, where $I(x)$ denotes the expected number of infections, given an HIV prevention investment of x dollars.

This model is easily extended to multiple interventions. For example, one could consider the change in the number of new infections associated with both a small-group counseling program for men who have sex with men and a large one-on-one outreach intervention for injection drug users. As above, the number of new infections prevented by investing x_k dollars in intervention k is $I_k(x_k) = I_k(0) - I_k(x_k)$, where I_k is the number of infections expected despite spending x_k dollars on the intervention. The total number of infections averted by a collection of n different interventions is:

$$A(x_1,x_2,\ldots,x_n) = \Delta I_1(x_1) + \Delta I_2(x_2) + \ldots + \Delta I_n(x_n). \quad (1)$$

Notice that the total spending associated with this resource allocation scheme is $x_1 + x_2 + \ldots + x_n$ dollars. Hence, if the total funds available for spending on HIV interventions equals B dollars, then the resource allocation scheme is affordable only if

$$x_1 + x_2 + \ldots + x_n \leq B. \quad (2)$$

Kaplan's model provides a procedure for maximizing the number of infections averted by a collection of n interventions, $A(x_1,x_2,\ldots,x_n)$, subject to the budgetary constraint given in equation 2. The output of the model is a specification of the ideal funding levels x_1, x_2, ..., x_n for the n interventions that would produce the greatest reduction in the number of new infections.

This basic model does not directly incorporate political or equity concerns but calculates the maximum number of infections that can be averted given an overall budget constraint. On occasion, political or social gains may justify a reduction in the optimal number of prevented infections. Kaplan[9] demonstrates how under certain circumstances, political, social, or other concerns can be added to the model in the form of additional constraints as well as how to calculate the "efficiency loss" associated with the additional constraint. For example, for reasons of equity, a CPG might want to ensure that each of three interventions receive at least c dollars. This could be accomplished by imposing the constraint: $x_i \geq c$ ($i = 1,2,3$). To estimate the efficiency loss, the basic model (described above) is run to determine the optimal allocation scheme given the new constraint. The number of infections that would be averted by the new, constrained allocation scheme then is compared to the number that would be averted by the optimal scheme to determine the efficiency loss. For example, if the optimal number of infections were 45 and the socially constrained number of infections were 43, then the efficiency loss would be equal to two infections or 4.4 percent. Is it better to attain equity by having all groups receive at least c dollars and to sacrifice two preventable infections, or to opt for the optimal number of cases prevented, excluding any equity considerations? The answer is subjective and is likely to vary across CPGs.

To implement this model requires that the CPG members obtain estimates of the main parameters, I(0) and I(x). Kaplan[9] proposes several methods that could be used to determine reasonable estimates of these parameters, most of which would require the CPG to seek the assistance of trained epidemiologists, health department experts, or local researchers. HIV incidence studies provide one source of estimates for the number of infections that would be expected if there were no interventions, I(0).[38,39] However, relatively few such studies have been conducted that can provide local information for use by CPGs. Recently, Holmberg[40] derived prevalence and incidence estimates for the 96 largest metropolitan statistical areas in the U.S. based on an extensive review of the published literature and other sources of information. The number of new infections over time also can be estimated using a statistical method known as backcalculation, in which HIV incidence rates are estimated from AIDS incidence data by backcalculating the estimated date of onset of HIV infection.[41] Although the incidence rates obtained by backcalculation techniques are not exact, this technique can provide an estimate of the rate of new infections when there are no other means available.

Few studies have attempted to measure the number of infections averted by HIV prevention interventions and those that typically have done so were within the context of assessing the cost-effectiveness of the target interventions.[4,42,43] Kaplan[9] also suggested a technique that entails subjectively constructing a link between infections averted and cost. CPGs start with a fixed budget and discuss what they think the likely impact of spending a particular amount of money on a particular intervention would be on the number of new infections resulting from implementing the intervention. Technically, however, CPGs prioritize but the health department allocates resources. The software is available through electronic mail (e-mail) from the author (Ed Kaplan, edward.kaplan@yale.edu); it requires Microsoft Excel (Windows '95 version or higher). Although this method has been pilot tested, it has not, to our knowledge, been adopted for regular use by any CPG.

Utility-based prioritization method

The general idea of the ranking method—that each person should rate each intervention or at risk population on multiple criteria—can be extended to take into account the subjective importance of each of the criteria. (For simplicity, we will describe the application of this method to the problem of prioritizing interventions (see Appendix 1)). In this scheme, criteria that the CPG believes are important are given greater weight than those it feels are less important.

This method is proposed here for the first time. It is derived from the decision-theoretic evaluation field[8] and it has been applied in decision analysis with multiple objectives: for example, in the context of deciding where to build the Mexico city airport.[44] For more recent references using this method and for citation of its assessment, see above.

There are four main steps in the process, which is based on MAUT.

1. Decide on a set of criteria—some of which might be very important and some of which might be much less important on which the interventions will be judged (examples include expected effectiveness, sustainability, community acceptance, feasibility, and so forth).

2. Assign "importance" weights to the different criteria to reflect the subjective judgment of the CPG regarding how much influence these criteria should have in the decision-making process.
3. Rate each intervention on how well it meets each criterion (for example, how sustainable is it?).
4. Combine weights and ratings into overall scores and rank (i.e., prioritize) the interventions based on these scores.

Although this method is complex, it is easily automated (a Microsoft Excel spreadsheet is being developed by the lead author, Johnson-Masotti). The required steps are described in greater detail below and are illustrated in Appendix 1.

The first step in applying the multiattribute utility model of prioritization is to determine relevant criteria on which to judge the interventions. This can be done through a group consensus method in which CPG members continue suggesting possible criteria until an exhaustive list has been compiled. The list then can be pared down by voting on whether each of the listed criteria should be retained or removed from the list. Remember that the criteria will be rated subsequently as to their importance so there is no need to remove all the less important criteria from the list at this stage. In fact, the only items that should be removed are those that are clearly irrelevant to the prioritization process (e.g., whether the intervention's name begins with "P"). Examples of potential criteria for ranking interventions include cost; expected or demonstrated effectiveness; scientific foundation; familiarity/past experience; acceptability to target communities; feasibility; legality; sustainability, and so forth.[5] In addition, we suggest adding a "personal preference" criterion that permits each CPG member to assign scores to the interventions based solely on his or her own subjective preferences. This is so that personal preferences are distinguished explicitly because they are inherent in any of the decision tools described herein. For purposes of illustration, suppose four criteria have been identified: C_1, C_2, C_3, and C_4.

Next, the importance weights for each criterion are determined (in the technical literature, these are known as "utilities"). The weights should be numbered between 0 and 1, with 1 representing an extremely important criterion and 0 representing a criterion that can be ignored completely. One of the most straightforward ways to accomplish this is to have each CPG member independently rank the criteria in terms of importance from most important to least important (e.g., C_2, C_4, C_1, C_3,). Each CPG member then should translate these rankings into weights that reflect the relative importance of the different criteria. The CPG member can do this by assigning a score of 1 to the criterion that he or she feels is the least important (criterion C_3 in this example) and then asking, "how much more important is criterion C_1 (the second least important one) than criterion C_3?" Similarly, "how much more important is criterion C_4 than criterion C_1?" and "how much more important is criterion C_2 than criterion C_4?" also should be asked. Simple arithmetic can be used to derive weights from the responses to these questions. For example, suppose a CPG member said that C_1 is twice as important as C_3; C_4 is one-and-one-half times as important as C_1; and C_2 is three times as important as C_4. Then, if one assigns a score of 1 to the least important criterion (C_3), one should assign scores of 2, 3, and 9, respectively, to criterion C_1, C_4, and C_2. The final step is to convert these to numbers between 0 and 1 by dividing each score by the sum of all the scores ($1 + 2 + 3 + 9 = 15$). The final weights for criterion C_1, C_2, C_3, and C_4 are then: $w_{C1} = 2/15$, $w_{C2} = 9/15$, $w_{C3} = 1/15$, and $w_{C4} = 3/15$.

In step three, each CPG member should assign a rating to each intervention for each of the criteria. The rating—a number between 0 and 100—should reflect the extent to which the intervention satisfies the criteria. For example, an unquestionably completely legal intervention should receive a rating of 100 on the "legality" criteria, whereas one that is banned by state or federal law should receive a rating of 0. Notice that this is very different from the previous step, in which CPG members judged the importance of the criteria themselves. In the present step, whether or not the criterion is important is inconsequential; all that matters is the extent to which the intervention meets the criterion. We suggest that CPG members assign these ratings on a criterion-by-criterion basis in order to facilitate comparisons of one intervention to another; for example, the member should assign "legality" ratings to all the interventions before moving on to the next criterion.

In the final step, the CPG members' importance weights and ratings are combined to derive an overall utility score for each intervention. Symbolically, the utility score assigned to intervention *i* by CPG member *j* is:

$$U_{ij} = \Sigma_k \, w_{jk} * r_{ijk} \quad (3)$$

where the sum is taken over the *k* different criteria; w_{jk} represents the importance weight assigned to criterion *k* by CPG member *j*; and r_{ijk} denotes the rating on criterion *k* that intervention *i* received from CPG member *j* (see the example in Appendix 1 for further clarification). The total utility score for the intervention is just the sum of the scores it received from the individual CPG members:

$$U_i = \Sigma_j \, U_{ij}. \quad (4)$$

At this stage of the procedure, each intervention has been assigned a utility score that reflects its priority ranking; thus, the highest priority intervention is the one with the largest utility score, the second highest priority goes to the intervention with the second greatest utility score, and so on.

Comparison of Methods

The four prioritization methods described above differ on a number of dimensions including ease of use, data requirements, range of potential responses, time required to implement the method, amount of work and number of people involved, opportunities for everyone to express their opinions, equal weighting of individuals' choices, and the likely acceptability of the method. It is expected that they also would differ on the "quality" of the rankings they produce. However, because there is no one goal of the prioritization process, it is difficult to define much less measure "quality." Table 1 summarizes the advantages and disadvantages of the four methods with regard to effectiveness, efficiency, equity, and political feasibility. In deciding which method to use, CPG members and others may use the following table to guide their selection of methods by determining which factors are most important to them, and comparing the available methods on these factors.

The ranking method is the simplest of the four methods. It does not require much information: once the criteria have been decided upon, no further information is needed. This procedure yields a limited response range (i.e., it does not permit fine distinctions to be drawn between the interventions or populations being prioritized). This method can be implemented fairly quickly once criteria have been chosen. Only one or two people are needed for gathering and totaling the scores given to the interventions or populations by the different CPG members. CPG members express their opinions at one level

Table 1

Comparison of four prioritization methods

		Alternatives			
Goals	**Criteria**	**Ranking**	**Holtgrave**	**Kaplan**	**Utility-based**
Precision	1. Permits fine distinctions between interventions or populations	low	moderate	low	moderate/high
Ease of use	1. Time	low	moderate/high	high	moderate/high
	2. Work involved	low	moderate	high	moderate
	3. Number of people involved	low	low	high	low/moderate
	4. Data requirements	low	moderate/high	high	moderate
Equity	1. Chance for everyone to express their opinions	low	moderate	moderate/high	high
	2. Equal weighting of individuals' choices	low	moderate	low	high
Political feasibility	1. Acceptability of methods and results to CPGs	high	moderate	low	moderate

only—by ranking interventions and populations; there is no room for expression of personal opinions or opportunity for expression of political affiliations. The likelihood for equal weighting of individuals' choices is high because a person's ranking is very likely to be similar to that of another person's. This method is likely to be acceptable to many CPGs because of its simplicity and ease of use.

Holtgrave's prioritization model is very practical and is the second least complex method of the four. It is not as simple to use as the ranking method, however, because it requires several additional steps beyond ranking interventions or populations. Also, more data are needed for this method such as numerical estimates of unmet needs and the number of potential infections that would occur if no intervention were implemented as well as estimates of the effectiveness of various interventions. The range of possible responses is limited because CPG members are asked to assign a narrow range of scores between zero and three. This method is more time consuming and it requires a larger amount or work than the ranking method because it entails a three-step process. Only a couple of individuals are needed, however, to agglomerate all scores. All CPG members have a chance to vote on the different steps of the process, but there is no room for expressing personal opinions. The likelihood for equal weighting of individuals' scores is moderate because scores are not standardized: for example, a person's total score may outweigh another person's, who may be circumspect. Acceptance by CPG members is enhanced by the detailed guidance available.[4]

Kaplan's model is very thorough but very complex as well. It is the most intensive of the four methods because it requires information on how many infections can be prevented by investing a given amount of money in a particular set of one or more HIV prevention interventions; and how many infections can be prevented by not investing any amount of money in any HIV intervention. This method can incorporate social constraints explicitly into the modeling process, giving CPG members a fair chance to express their opinions. The likelihood for equal weighting of CPG members' scores is small because somebody may stir production function values to his or her own satisfaction and values are not standardized. Alternatively, CPG members need to sell the production function to fellow members and any bias will have a lower chance of success. The response range is rather narrow. This method is the most difficult method of the four, it is very time consuming, it requires many iterations, and it necessitates the use of a computer. The scoring process may require more than two individuals. This method may be unacceptable to many CPGs because of its complexity.

Finally, the utility-based prioritization method is moderate to high in difficulty. This method requires little more data than the ranking method. Its main advantage is that it incorporates value judgments directly into the evaluation process. This method takes into account conflicting objectives, yielding information that is directly usable from the standpoint of decision makers. Scores given by CPG members are standardized, ensuring a high likelihood of equal and fair weighting on CPG members' choices. This method allows for the greatest range in responses but the time involved in implementing the method may be long as individuals give scores to criteria based on their preferences and assign ratings to each criterion. The amount of work needed to implement this method is greater than for the ranking method but probably not as great as for Kaplan's method. Somebody needs to enter into a computer the scores and ratings assigned by each CPG member. This method is likely to be acceptable to CPG members because it incorporates their value judgments; on the other hand, it is complex and may seem overly quantitative to some CPG members.

Discussion

This article describes in detail four methods that can be used by HIV prevention CPGs to aid in prioritizing population needs and interventions to address those needs. It also compares and contrasts these four methods in terms of effectiveness, efficiency, equity, and political feasibility.

Further research is needed on prioritization methods, with the ultimate goal of establishing a standardized technique that can be used by all CPGs but includes enough flexibility to allow for local adaptations. Methods such as the utility-based prioritization method presented here that allow for the inclusion of values and judgments appear to be the best suited for the difficult task faced by CPGs, which must make their decisions based on limited empirical data within a highly charged, political atmosphere. Past research indicates that CPG members often use value judgments, especially when data are unavailable. Therefore, methods that permit value judgments to be combined with empirical data could be especially appropriate for use in this context.

As a first step toward the development of a standardized method that is both acceptable and useful, promising candidates such as the utility-based prioritization method introduced above should be presented to CPGs "in the field" and their performance should be evaluated. As discussed in the preceding section, some of the most important attributes of a good prioritization method are ease of use, data requirements, range of response rates, time for implementing the method, amount of work involved, number of people involved, chance for everyone to express their opinions, likelihood of equal/fair weighting on individuals' choices, the likely acceptability of the method, and satisfaction with the outcome of the process. Existing prioritization techniques should be field tested and revised as needed to improve their performance.

Although it is too soon to know, it may not be possible to achieve the standardization envisioned here: a standardized, widely accepted, and theoretically sound method for algorithmically prioritizing interventions and populations. It may be that the issue of HIV prevention prioritization is inherently too contentious, too political, and too personal to be reduced to a series of simple steps. Nevertheless, the methods described above can still play an important role in the prioritization process by helping CPGs make their values and assumptions explicit. For example, a CPG might go through the utility-based procedure first as a nonbinding exercise to help members gauge the overall, groupwide importance of different criteria and to get a sense of how different interventions (or populations) rate on these criteria. The group then could proceed to use another method—perhaps even an informal one such as group consensus building—to arrive at the final prioritization list.

In the end, the methods presented here are simply decision tools. It is hoped that they can help guide the decision-making process in ways that are consistent with the goals of the CPG itself. HIV prevention planning is a very difficult task and any tool that makes it easier is indeed welcome.

REFERENCES

1. Centers for Disease Control and Prevention, "Cooperative Agreements for Human Immunodeficiency Virus (HIV) Prevention Projects, Intervention Announcement and Availability of Funds for the Fiscal Year 1993," *Federal Register* 57 (1992): 40675–40683.
2. D.R. Holtgrave and R.O. Valdiserri, "Year One of HIV Prevention Community Planning: A National Perspective on Accomplishments, Challenges, and Future Directions," *Journal of Public Health Management and Practice* 2, no. 3 (1996): 1–9.
3. R.O. Valdiserri, et al., "Community Planning: A National Strategy To Improve HIV Prevention Interventions," *Journal of Community Health* 20 (1995): 87–100.
4. D.R. Holtgrave, "Setting Priorities and Community Planning for HIV-Prevention Interventions," *AIDS & Public Policy Journal* 9 (1994): 145–151.
5. Academy for Education Development and National Alliance of State and Territorial AIDS Directors, *HIV Prevention Priorities: How Community Planning Groups Decide*. Atlanta: Centers for Disease Control and Prevention, 1996.
6. Academy for Educational Development and Centers for Disease Control, *Handbook for HIV Prevention Community Planning*. Washington, DC: Academy for Educational Development, 1994.
7. A.P. Johnson-Masotti, et al., "Decision Making in HIV Prevention Community Planning: An Integrative Review," *Journal of Community Health* 25, no 2(2000):95–112.
8. W.N. Dunn, *Public Policy Analysis—An Introduction*. Englewood Cliffs, NJ: Prentice Hall, 1994.
9. E.H. Kaplan, "Economic Evaluation and HIV Prevention Community Planning: A Policy Analyst's Perspective," in *Handbook of Economic Evaluation of HIV Prevention Interventions*, ed. D.R. Holtgrave. New York and London: Plenum, 1998.
10. Centers for Disease Control and Prevention, *HIV Prevention Community Planning: Shared Decision Making in Action*. Atlanta: Centers for Disease Control and Prevention, 1998.
11. Centers for Disease Control and Prevention, *External Review of FY 97 HIV Prevention Continuation Applications and Comprehensive HIV Prevention Plans—Summary of Process and Findings*. Atlanta: Centers for Disease Control and Prevention, 1997.
12. Centers for Disease Control and Prevention, *APEXPH: Assessment Protocol for Excellence in Public Health*. Atlanta: U.S. Department of Health and Human Services, 1991.
13. A.D. Spiegel and H.H. Human, *Basic Health Planning Methods*. Germantown, MD: Aspen Systems Corp, 1978.
14. J.J. Hanlon, "The Design of Public Health Programs for Underdeveloped Countries," *Public Health Reports* 69 (1954): 1028.
15. T.O. Tengs, et al., "Oregon's Medicaid Ranking and Cost-Effectiveness: Is There Any Relationship?" *Medical Decision Making* 16, no. 2 (1996): 99–107.

16. A. Bowling, "Health Care Rationing: The Public's Debate," *British Medical Journal* 312, no. 7032 (1996): 670–674.
17. W.T. Sanderson, et al., "Pesticide Prioritization for a Brain Cancer Case-Control Study," *Environmental Research* 74, no. 2 (1997): 133–144.
18. J.S. Seidel, et al., "Priorities for Research in Emergency, Medical Services for Children: Results of a Consensus Conference," *Pediatric Emergency Care* 15, no. 1 (1999): 55–58.
19. J.M. Harrington and I.A. Calvert, "Research Priorities in Occupational Medicine: A Survey of United Kingdom Personnel Managers," *Occupational & Environmental Medicine* 53, no. 9 (1996): 642–644.
20. S. Senn, "Some Statistical Issues in Project Prioritization in the Pharmaceutical Industry," *Statistics in Medicine* 14, no. 24 (1996): 2689–2702.
21. S. Dixon, et al., "The Application of Evidence-Based Priority Setting in District Health Authority," *Journal of Public Health Medicine* 19, no. 3 (1997): 307–312.
22. J.A. Olsen, "Aiding Priority Setting in Health Care: Is There a Role for the Contingent Valuation Method?" *Health Economics* 6, no. 6 (1997): 603–612.
23. U.S. Conference of Mayors, *HIV Prevention Community Planning Profiles: Assessing Year One*. Washington, DC: U.S. Conference of Mayors, 1995.
24. S.F. Spear, et al., "Cost-Utility Assessment: Planning with Local Decision-Makers in Developing Countries," *Public Administration and Development* 8 (1988): 457–465.
25. P. Reagan-Cirincione and J. Rohrbaugh, "Decision Conferencing: A Unique Approach to the Behavioral Aggregation of Expert Judgement," in *Expertise and Decision Support*, ed. G. Wright and F. Bolger. New York: Plenum, 1992.
26. C.A. Bellamy, et al., "Measurement of Patient-Delivered Utility Values for Periodontal Health Using Multi-Attribute Scale," *Journal of Clinical Periodontology* 23, no. 9 (1996): 805–809.
27. W.C. Lin and C. Ball, "Factors Affecting the Decision of Nursing Students in Taiwan To Be Vaccinated against Hepatitis B Infection," *Journal of Advanced Nursing* 25, no. 4 (1997): 709–718.
28. V. Lawson, et al., "The Family Impact of Childhood Atopic Dermatitis: The Dermatitis Family Impact Questionnaire," *British Journal of Dermatology* 138, no. 1 (1998): 107–113.
29. R.W. Shaw, et al., "Perceptions of Women on the Impact of Menorrhagia on Their Health Using Multi-Attribute Utility Assessment," *British Journal of Obstetrics & Gynaecology* 105, no. 11 (1998): 1155–1159.
30. P.J. Neumann, et al., "Health Utilities in Alzheimer's Disease: A Cross-Sectional Study of Patients and Caregivers," *Medical Care* 37, no. 1 (1999): 27–32.
31. D. Timmermans and C. Vlek, "Effects on Decision Quality of Supporting Multi-Attribute Evaluation in Groups," *Organizational Behavior & Human Decision Processes* 68, no. 2 (1996): 158–170.
32. H. Pollack and R. Zeckhauser, "Budgets as Dynamic Gatekeepers," *Management Science* 42 (1996): 642–658.
33. M.E. Cowen, et al., "A Guide for Planning Community-Oriented Health Care: The Health Sector Resource Allocation Model," *Medical Care* 34, no. 3 (1996): 264–279.
34. S. Kim, et al., "Algorithms for Resource Allocation of Substance Abuse Prevention Funds Based on the Estimated Need: A Case Study on State of Florida—Part 1," *Journal of Drug Education* 28, no. 2 (1998): 87–106.
35. J. Blalock and P.A. Mackowiak, "A Resource-Allocation Model To Enhance Productivity of Academic Physicians," *Academic Medicine* 73, no. 10 (1998): 1062–1066.
36. S. Kim, et al., "Algorithms for Resource Allocation of Substance Abuse Prevention Funds Based on the Estimated Need: A Case Study on State of Florida—Part 2," *Journal of Drug Education* 28, no. 3 (1998): 169–184.
37. E.H. Kaplan and H. Pollack, "Allocating HIV Prevention Resources," *Socio-Economic Planning Sciences* 32 (1998): 257–263.
38. R. Brookmeyer and T.C. Quinn, "Estimation of Current Human Immunodeficiency Virus Incidence Rates from a Cross-Sectional Survey Using Early Diagnostic Tests," *American Journal of Epidemiology* 141 (1995): 166–172.
39. E.H. Kaplan and R. Brookmeyer, "Snapshot Estimators of Recent HIV Incidence Rates," *Operations Research* 47 (1999): 29–37.
40. S.D. Holmberg, "The Estimated Prevalence and Incidence of HIV in 96 Large U.S. Metropolitan Areas," *American Journal of Public Health* 86 (1996): 642–654.
41. R. Brookmeyer and M.H. Gail, *AIDS Epidemiology: A Quantitative Approach*. Oxford: Oxford University Press, 1994.
42. D.R. Holtgrave, et al., "Quantitative Economic Evaluations of HIV-Related Prevention and Treatment Services: A Review," *Risk* 5 (1994): 29–47.
43. D.R. Holtgrave, et al., "Effectiveness and Efficiency of HIV Prevention Services: An Overview," *Public Health Reports* 110 (1995): 134–146.
44. R.L. Keeney, "A Decision Analysis with Multiple Objectives: The Mexico City Airport," *Bell Journal of Economics and Management Science* 4 (1973): 101–117.

Appendix 1

Utility-Based Prioritization Model

Suppose that in Step 1 the CPG identified four criteria (C_1, C_2, C_3, and C_4) to be used in ranking three Interventions (I_1, I_2, and I_3).

Step #2: Assign importance weights to criteria.

Substep 2.1: Rank the criteria from most important to least important

Most important: C_2
C_4
C_1
Least important: C_3

Substep 2.2: Judge how much more important C_1 is than C_3; C_4 is than C_1; and C_2 is than C_4

C_1 is 2 times as important as C_3 [$C_1 = 2*C_3$]
C_4 is 1.5 times as important as C_1 [$C_4 = 1.5*C_1$]
C_2 is 3 times as important as C_4 [$C_2 = 3*C_4$]

Substep 2.3: Assign the least important criterion an importance score of 1 and calculate importance scores for other criteria using relationships from Substep 2.1

$C_3 = 1$
$C_1 = 2*C_3 = 2$
$C_4 = 1.5*C_1 = 3$
$C_2 = 3*C_4 = 9$

Substep 2.4: Sum the importance scores and divide each score by the sum to obtain the importance weights, which are numbers between 0 and 1

$\text{Sum} = C_1 + C_2 + C_3 + C_4 = 2 + 9 + 1 + 3 = 15$
$w_{j1} = C_1/\text{Sum} = 2/15$
$w_{j2} = C_2/\text{Sum} = 9/15$
$w_{j3} = C_3/\text{Sum} = 1/15$
$w_{j4} = C_4/\text{Sum} = 3/15$
(The subscript *j* indicates that these are the weights assigned to the criteria by CPG member *j*)

Step #3: Rate each intervention on the basis of each criterion

Substep 3.1: First rate each intervention on the basis of criterion 1

Intervention 1: $r_{1j1} = 25$
Intervention 2: $r_{2j1} = 100$
Intervention 3: $r_{3j1} = 80$
(The first and third subscripts indicate the intervention and criteria, respectively, while the subscript *j* indicates that these ratings were assigned by CPG member j)

Substep 3.2: Now rate each intervention on the basis of criteria 2, 3, and then 4

Intervention 1: $r_{1j2} = 16$; $r_{1j3} = 0$; $r_{1j4} = 40$
Intervention 2: $r_{2j2} = 12$; $r_{2j3} = 10$; $r_{2j4} = 50$
Intervention 3: $r_{3j2} = 93$; $r_{3j3} = 63$; $r_{3j4} = 28$

Step #4: Calculate overall utility of each intervention and prioritize interventions

Substep 4.1: Calculate utility assigned to intervention *i* by CPG member *j*

$U_{ij} = \sum k\ w_{jk} * r_{ijk}$
Intervention 1: $U_{1j} = w_{j1}*r_{1j1} + w_{j2}*r_{1j2} + w_{j3}*r_{1j3} + w_{j4}*r_{1j4} = 20.93$
Intervention 2: $U_{1j} = w_{j1}*r_{2j1} + w_{j2}*r_{2j2} + w_{j3}*r_{2j3} + w_{j4}*r_{2j4} = 31.20$
Intervention 3: $U_{1j} = w_{j1}*r_{3j1} + w_{j2}*r_{3j2} + w_{j3}*r_{3j3} + w_{j4}*r_{3j4} = 76.27$

Substep 4.2:	Calculate overall utility for intervention *i* $U_1 = \Sigma_j U_{ij}$ (This step requires summing the overall utility scores for intervention *i* assigned to it by each of the CPG members. The above example considers only a single CPG member, hence it is not possible to carry this example further)
Substep 4.3:	Prioritize interventions in order of the overall utility scores calculated in Substep 4.2

Assessing the HIV Prevention Capacity Building Needs of Community-Based Organizations

Donna L. Richter, Mary S. Prince, Linda H. Potts, Belinda M. Reininger, Melva V. Thompson, Jacquie P. Fraser, and Susan L. Fulmer

Community-based organizations (CBOs) have been providing HIV prevention services to priority populations for many years. Recent research suggests that CBOs could benefit from capacity building to strengthen their public health prevention knowledge and skills, including ability to access and use behavioral science to guide prevention efforts. A cross-sectional survey of 316 CBOs was conducted to assess desire and preferences for training, support for training at the organizational level, motivation for training at the individual level, barriers to training, and factors associated with the perceived need for training. Results suggest the need for a national training initiative to increase CBO capacity.

Introduction

In 1997, the Centers for Disease Control and Prevention (CDC) provided a total of $18 million in direct funding to community-based organizations (CBOs) through Program Announcement 704.[1] As in

This project was funded under ASPH/CDC/ATSDR Cooperative Agreement S700 18/18.

Donna L. Richter, EdD, *is the Chair of the Department of Health Promotion and Education in the School of Public Health at the University of South Carolina, Columbia, South Carolina.*

Mary S. Prince, PhD, *is the President of Health Promotion Works in Pawleys Island, South Carolina and adjunct faculty at the Rollins School of Public Health at Emory University, Atlanta, Georgia.*

Linda H. Potts, MPH, MBA, *is the President of Health Consulting Group, Inc. in Atlanta, Georgia.*

Belinda M. Reininger, DrPH, *is an Assistant Professor in the Department of Health Promotion and Education in the School of Public Health at the University of South Carolina in Columbia, South Carolina.*

Melva V. Thompson, DrPH, *is a Post Doctoral Fellow in the Department of Health Promotion and Education in the School of Public Health at the University of South Carolina, Columbia, South Carolina.*

Jacquie P. Fraser, PhD, *is an Assistant Professor at Armstrong Atlantic State University in Savannah, Georgia.*

Susan L. Fulmer, MPH, MS, *is Program Manager/ Assistant Director of the SC AIDS Training Network in Columbia, South Carolina.*

the past, the recipients of direct funding initiatives were mandated to develop and implement effective community-based human immunodeficiency virus (HIV) prevention programs and promote collaboration and coordination of HIV prevention efforts with other organizations in their community. However, recent research suggests CBOs may not possess all the requisite skills needed to fulfill these requirements. To increase the prevention capacity of CBOs, the CDC contracted with the Association of the Schools of Public Health and the Department of Health Promotion in the School of Public Health at the University of South Carolina to assess the possibility of implementing a national training program in HIV prevention for CBO program managers. A national survey of 517 CBOs was conducted to assess program managers' desire, needs, and preferences for HIV prevention training. If the responding CBOs expressed an interest in participating in a national training program, data from the survey would be used to design a training model targeted to increase the HIV prevention capacity of CBO program managers.

Background

An evaluation of HIV prevention programs in nine high-prevalence cities in 1984 led the CDC to the following conclusion: for HIV/acquired immune deficiency syndrome (AIDS) prevention programs to be effective, they needed to be culturally appropriate and involve multiple players.[2] One of the principal players identified as being essential in the fight against the spread of HIV was community-based organizations.[2–5] Originally formed to fill the gap in services reaching those populations most in need, CBOs consistently have served as frontline providers of HIV prevention programs since the emergence of the epidemic in 1981.

But as the epidemic persists, the strategies required to implement an effective prevention program have become more involved. Do CBOs possess the skills needed to keep up with the latest technologies for minimizing the incidence of HIV?

Translating effective intervention from the research setting to the community setting has proved challenging as the skills needed to effectively tailor successful research interventions into programs addressing the needs of a specific community are complex. To unravel the psychological, social, cultural, and economic elements influencing the spread of HIV, contributions from all the social and behavioral disciplines were required.[6] The components of a successful prevention program now include: examining data on the epidemic in specific target populations; accessing and understanding current behavioral research and theory; selecting behavioral factors to target; reviewing the literature to see what interventions worked to change which behaviors in a specific population; shaping the intervention to the cultural, social, and political environment of the target population; and conducting process and outcome evaluations to measure change resulting from the intervention.[7] Even for seasoned professionals, these tasks are challenging and research suggests that CBOs may lack the requisite skills to effectively assess and use the behavioral science techniques and strategies that are proving to be successful.

In 1996, the CDC and the Academy for Educational Development requested a team of scientists from the American Psychological Association to peruse evaluations prepared by the CDC and seven external evaluators to determine the unmet needs of HIV Community Planning Groups (CPGs). In most communities, CBOs are active partners in their local CPG. The objective of the evaluation was to measure the use of behavioral science and behavioral science techniques in HIV prevention planning. The investigators were especially interested in determining CPGs' ability to gather epidemiological data on the targeted community, conduct needs assessments, prioritize needs, and match behavioral theory with necessary action. After examining all of the evaluation materials collectively, the scientists found CPGs lacking in their ability to access and use behavioral science to guide their prevention efforts.[8]

Additional research specifically on CBOs supported the conclusions of Sparks and her colleagues. A survey of 25 CBOs in San Francisco found that, while most CBOs had used strategies from behavioral research in the past, many lacked the time and resources to access it efficiently.[9] This study also found that translating behavioral science literature into program application as well as simply understanding the language of the behavioral scientists challenged most CBO staff. The language and methods used to describe research interventions are not the vocabulary of CBOs and little help exists to translate findings into more meaningful expressions.

A national survey of CBO program managers also found funding and time as barriers to accessing behavioral information for prevention planning.[10] CBOs were more likely to use their peers from other CBOs as their most important source of information rather than relying on research publications, scientific conferences, or collaborating with behavioral science researchers to inform their HIV prevention planning.

The concept of behavioral capability contends that for a person to perform a new behavior, he or she must know what a behavior is (knowledge) and how to perform it (skill).[11] Following this logic, CBOs need access to behavioral research (knowledge) and practice at adapting the techniques that are identified in the behavioral literature as being critical to HIV prevention practice (skill). Training can develop both of these competencies. However, training has not always been rated highly by CBOs.[8,10] Therefore, if training is to be an effective means of bridging the gap between research and practice for CBOs, the training model needs to be tailored to the needs and preferences of CBO HIV prevention program managers.

Methodology

Study purpose and design

The principal purpose for this investigation was to develop a training model with a public health focus in HIV/AIDS prevention that is appropriate for CBO program managers. Six areas of inquiry were explored in the survey: (1) desire for training, (2) organizational support for training, (3) benefits of attending training program, (4) barriers to attending training program, (5) preferred topics for training, and (6) preferred format for training.

The study was designed to measure the difference in training needs of HIV/AIDS prevention and education program managers across different categories of CBOs. Two particular groups of interest were CDC-funded (direct) CBOs and nonCDC-funded CBOs. These two groups were chosen based on the limited literature regarding the impact of funding on CBOs and their training needs. The study used a cross-sectional survey design to capture potential variation in training needs and preferences.

Methods

Population sampled

The population sample for this study was all CBOs that at the time of the survey were either (1) currently funded by the CDC for HIV/AIDS prevention activities or (2) seeking funding under CDC Program Announcement 704. By default, because of eligibility requirements for CDC funding, respondents also were (1) tax-exempt, nonprofit CBOs with an established record of service and (2) had plans to develop at least one Health Education and Risk Reduction program for HIV prevention in 1998. Additional characteristics of the CBOs within the selected sample included being primarily minority (67%) and serving high-prevalence areas (84%). To be designated a minority CBO, ethnic or racial minorities needed to compose 51 percent or more of the CBO's board of directors. CBOs from 47 states (Indiana, New Hampshire, North Dakota excluded), the District of Columbia, and three U.S. territories (Guam, Pohnpei, Puerto Rico) were represented in the sample.

Instrumentation

A seven-member advisory board was established to assist in developing the survey instrument. The board was composed of representatives from three CDC-funded CBOs, two nonCDC-funded CBOs, one representative from the National and Regional Minority Organizations, and one representative from a state health department. Geographical areas of the country also were represented by membership. The role of the board was to provide input into the design of the survey by identifying the following: (1) variables classifying CBOs, (2) factors thought to motivate participation, (3) factors thought to be possible barriers to training, (4) desired content areas for training, and (5) areas of cultural sensitivity.

CBO representatives on the advisory board and representatives from three additional CBOs participated in the pilot test of the survey instrument. Each participant was mailed a survey along with an accompanying cover letter that explained how the respondents should proceed. Also, a survey critique sheet was mailed with the survey and respondents were asked to complete and return this form as well. The recommended changes provided by respondents were incorporated and the revised instrument was mailed to members of the advisory board for final review, comment, and approval.

The survey instrument was prepared in booklet form. It was an eight-page, 95-item questionnaire. Twenty-two items assessed CBO "demographic" characteristics and five multiple-item scales were used to measure the dependent variables of interest: organizational support, incentives for training, barriers to training, topics for training, and preferred formats for training.

Procedure

A modified version of Dillman's Total Design Method[12] for mailed surveys was followed to help ensure a maximum response rate. Prior to mailing out the survey, the CDC was asked to notify funded CBOs about the survey and its importance. One week following CDC notification, surveys were mailed to the executive directors of all CBOs. Each packet mailed contained a cover letter explaining what the survey was about and the usefulness of the survey, a questionnaire, and reply envelope. Ten days following the first mailing, a reminder postcard was sent out to all nonrespondents asking them to return their completed instruments. Two weeks later, a trained team of callers started contacting nonrespondents by telephone asking them to return their completed instruments, or if needed, obtaining the necessary information to ship a new questionnaire to them immediately. One hundred and seventy-three survey packets were re-shipped upon request. Five attempts were made to contact the CBO executive director or program manager before the CBO was dropped from the study. After two months, nonresponding organizations were contacted again and surveys either were completed over the telephone or by Fax machine.

Analysis

Data were analyzed using SPSS-PC. Frequencies, means, and standard deviations were calculated on the data from all respondents, and outliers (SD > 2) that may have identified any undetected data entry errors or extremes in responses were examined and removed. Respondents then were categorized according to their funding status (CDC-funded and nonCDC-funded) and responses were analyzed for possible differences between the two groups with respect to their training needs and preferences for HIV prevention. To test for possible differences between CDC-funded CBOs and nonCDC-funded CBOs, the Chi square test was used for categorical dependent variables and one-way ANOVA was used for continuous dependent variables. All tests were considered significant at the .05 level. However, in order to analyze the differences between CDC-funded and nonCDC-funded CBOs, the five multiple-item scales measuring the dependent variables of interest, which included 11 to 15 items per scale, needed to be reduced. Factor analysis was used to reduce the number of items in each scale. The new factors were identified using eigenvalues, scree plot, and pattern matrix. Promax, an oblique rotation method, was used to redefine the initial factor solution for all scales. Only factors with loadings ≥ .45 were included in the analysis. Factor values were calculated using factor-based scores (mean sums).

Results

The results of this survey are presented as follows. Table 1 lists key characteristics of all responding CBOs. Tables 2–6 list the total mean scores of all respondents to all of the survey questions addressing training needs and preferences. A brief discussion of these results precedes each table. Table 7 shows the underlying factors that emerged from the factor analysis on the items that comprise Tables 2–6 and the results of the analysis comparing the responses of CDC-funded CBOs and nonCDC-funded CBOs. The CBO's executive director answered survey questions addressing organizational support for training and preferred length of training. All other areas of inquiry were directed to HIV prevention program managers. Understandably, in a small CBO, one person could fill both positions.

Description of the Sample

There were 517 CBOs included in the population sample, of which 84 were currently CDC-funded CBOs and 433 were new applicants for funding. (Any duplication of CBOs between the two groups was eliminated as currently funded CBOs seeking new funding were treated as "currently funded" only.) A total of 316 surveys were returned for an overall response rate of 61 percent. Seventy percent of CDC-funded CBOs returned completed questionnaires and 60 percent of nonCDC-funded CBOs responded. Key HIV prevention program characteristics of the 316 responding CBOs are reported in Table 1. CBOs' executive directors provided these data.

Table 1

Characteristics of sample

Key characteristics	CDC funded		NonCDC-funded		Total	
	N	%	N	%	N	%
Number of years providing prevention services						
0–3 years	1	2	69	27	70	23
4–10 years	47	85	146	57	193	62
Less than 10 years	7	13	41	16	48	15
Total	55	100	256	100	311	100
Location of CBOs						
Urban	48	89	189	74	237	77
Rural	1	2	15	6	16	5
Urban and rural	5	9	50	20	55	18
Total	54	100	254	100	308	100
Size of population served						
Less than 50,000	6	11	38	15	44	14
50,000–499,999	18	33	98	39	116	38
500,000–3,000,000	20	37	87	34	107	35
Greater than 3,000,000	10	19	31	12	41	13
Total	54	100	254	100	308	100
Ethnicity of target populations served						
African American	22	40	140	57	162	51
Hispanic/Latino	17	31	45	17	62	20
Caucasian	2	4	35	13	37	12
Other	14	25	41	16	53	17
Total	55	100	261	100	306	100
Target clients served						
Youth, in general	9	16	57	22	66	22
Men who have sex with men	11	20	53	20	64	21
Community at large	5	9	44	17	49	16
IVDUs	7	13	29	11	36	12
Women who have sex with men	7	13	28	11	35	11
Other	10	29	50	19	71	18
Total	55	100	261	100	306	100
Primary services provided						
Peer-based intervention	12	22	38	15	50	18
Risk reduction counseling	7	12	31	12	38	13
Street/bar outreach	8	15	28	11	36	13
Clinical services	5	9	24	9	30	10
Prevention case management	8	15	19	7	27	10
Other	15	27	111	43	102	36
Total	55	100	261	100	282	100

Training preferences and needs

Desire for training

More than 80 percent of all program managers felt they could use additional training in HIV prevention (data not shown), suggesting program managers would attend training if it was offered. There was no difference between program managers from CDC-funded CBOs and nonCDC-funded CBOs in their desire for training (Chi square = 1.000, p = .317).

Table 2

Organizational support for training ranked by mean score (range of scores: 4 = extremely likely to 1 = not likely)

Assuming program managers participate in an effective public health HIV/AIDS prevention training and share new knowledge and skills with your CBO, how likely would this result in:	Mean Score
Enhancing your CBO's ability to achieve desired outcomes of prevention programs	3.510
Enhancing your CBO's willingness to develop partnerships with other community groups to enhance program effectiveness	3.487
Assisting your CBO in identifying issues, strengths, and challenges in your organization's delivery of prevention programs	3.479
Enhancing your CBO's understanding of the strategies necessary to deliver effective prevention programs	3.464
Enhancing your CBO's ability to obtain future funding	3.436
Enhancing your CBO's ability to identify root causes and patterns promoting and impeding your prevention efforts	3.362
Enhancing the willingness of your CBO to test prevention theories and strategies new to your organization	3.350
Enhancing the willingness of your CBO to collect data for evaluation and planning	3.309
Facilitating the formation of participatory and cooperative teams, composed of your CBO's staff, to plan programs and solve problems	3.285
Enhancing your CBO's ability to ensure program maintenance after current funding ends	3.278
No changes because your CBO as a whole is too burdened with other services to alter your prevention program	1.565

Table 3

Benefits of attending training sessions according to prevention program managers ranked by mean score (range of scores: 4 = extremely important to 1 = not important)

Assuming all training-related costs were paid for you, how important would each of the following incentives be in your decision to attend HIV/AIDS prevention program training?	Mean Score
Ability to do my job better	3.761
Improving the overall prevention effectiveness of the CBO	3.755
Improving my ability to make purposeful choices when designing prevention strategies	3.729
Networking with other participants	3.478
Having time to discuss current issues with peers	3.453
Training would be re-energizing	3.400
Being given paid time off work to attend training	3.263
Supervisor encouragement	3.164
Receiving credits toward a degree	2.618
Receiving continuing education credits	2.603
Clarifying my personal reasons for choosing to work in HIV/AIDS prevention	2.578
Receiving a certificate of attendance	2.345
Documentation in my personnel file	2.213

Table 4

Barriers to attending training programs ranked by mean score (range of scores: 4 = strongly agree to 1 = strongly disagree)

Assuming training costs are not an issue, would the following influence your decision not to attend HIV/AIDS prevention training?	Mean Score
I could not attend without paid leave	2.938
If the training requires too much time away from my job, I would not be able to attend	2.793
I do not have access to downlink sites for satellite conferencing	2.665
There is no one to replace me and do my job while I am away	2.476
If the training requires too much time away from home, I would not want to participate	2.375
I am not able to do my job and a self-study course	1.890
I do not have access to computers and software for computerized training courses	1.801
I don't feel I need additional training in HIV/AIDS prevention	1.749
I don't feel there are sufficient incentives or rewards for me to participate in this type of training	1.739
I don't feel my new prevention ideas would be implemented in my CBO	1.631
I would be concerned about losing my job if I were gone for long periods of time	1.607
I don't feel this type of training is applicable to my job	1.563

Table 5

Preferred topics for training by prevention program managers ranked by mean score (range of scores: 4 = extremely likely to 1 = not likely)

Assuming there are no barriers to your participation, how likely would you be to participate in HIV/AIDS training in each of the following areas:	Mean Score
How to evaluate the effectiveness of HIV/AIDS prevention programs	3.640
How to use prevention data to improve prevention programs	3.638
How to empower/mobilize individuals and communities to prevent HIV/AIDS	3.570
How to determine what influences certain kinds of behavior and what causes people to behave in ways that put themselves at risk	3.562
How to assess a specific population's attitudes, beliefs, knowledge, and behavior related to HIV/AIDS	3.465
How to use assessment data to improve prevention programs	3.455
How to access and apply research findings to effectively plan, implement, and evaluate prevention programs	3.410
How to advocate for HIV/AIDS prevention resources	3.383
How to structure program activities to best fit your CBO's mission in HIV/AIDS prevention	3.367
How to implement and manage HIV/AIDS prevention programs	3.342
How to determine the cost-effectiveness of prevention program activities	3.334
How to plan and budget HIV/AIDS prevention programs	3.277
How to build community coalitions and community networks	3.246
How to conduct a community needs assessment	3.238
How to identify and collaborate with researchers and/or clinicians to assist in developing prevention programs	3.232

Table 6

Preferred formats for training ranked by mean score (range of scores: 4 = extremely likely to 1 = not likely)

How likely would you be to attend training offered in the following formats:	Mean Score
Workshops (one long session)	3.549
Seminar series (several short sessions)	3.416
On-the-job training	3.372
On-campus/in-classroom studies	3.062
A combination of in-classroom course and distance learning	2.885
Videotape self-studies	2.794
Computer-based self-study	2.721
Print-based self-study	2.603
Live satellite conferences	2.409
Internet/on-line electronic conferencing	2.403
Satellite conferences with self-study materials	2.400
Audio cassette self-studies	2.367
Telephone conference calls	2.341

Table 7

Differences between CDC-funded CBOs and nonCDC-funded CBOs across the following areas of inquiry: support for training at the organizational level, the benefits of training, barriers to training, preferred topics for training, preferred formats for training, preferred educational level of courses, and preferred length of training

	N		Mean		Std. deviation			
	F	NF	F	NF	F	NF	F	p
Organizational support								
Innovation	54	252	3.42	3.38	.516	.445	.390	.533
Maintenance	53	255	3.44	3.38	.573	.575	.416	.519
Benefits of training								
Personal rewards	54	252	2.59	2346	.730	.871	.996	.319
Stimulation	54	253	3.58	3.56	.428	.465	.071	.790
Barriers to training								
Separation	53	251	2.80	2.62	.562	.629	.355	.061
Convenience	53	251	2.02	2.10	.680	.639	.716	.398
Application	53	250	1.53	1.67	.476	.563	.416	.519
Preferred topics								
Topics	54	255	3.41	3.41	.502	.522	.008	.931
Preferred formats								
Distant	51	253	2.54	2.52	.612	.690	.044	.834
Personal Interaction	51	252	3.28	3.25	.477	.504	.113	.737
Preferred educational level								
Ed level	51	248	2.31	2.21	.62	.62	1.10	.834
Preferred length								
Length	53	247	1.77	1.96	.95	1.22	1.13	.288

Note: F = CDC-funded CBO; NF = nonCDC-funded CBO.

Organizational support for training

Training as a whole is an activity that is seen as worthwhile and beneficial to CBOs by their executive directors (see Table 2). They believe training is very likely to enhance their CBO's ability to achieve not only their organization's prevention objectives but also to increase their CBO's capacity to interact with other service organizations in their area, thereby affecting prevention efforts at the community level. Training will help accomplish this by helping program managers (1) identify their organization's internal strengths and weaknesses and (2) by increasing their understanding of effective strategies and models for preventing HIV/AIDS.

Benefits of attending a training program

Incentives or rewards of attending a training program are listed in Table 3. The results show that the desired benefits of training are altruistic. Prevention program managers see improving prevention programs and the overall effectiveness of the CBO as more important than receiving certification, credit, or documentation in their personnel file. The top three incentives for attending HIV/AIDS prevention training are the "ability to do my job better," "improving the overall effectiveness of the CBO," and "improving my ability to make purposeful choices."

Barriers to attending training program

Table 4 ranks the barriers to attending training programs. The most frequently cited reason for not attending a training program is that the training requires too much time away from the job (35.9%). Having to spend too much time away from home and not having a replacement on the job while the trainee is away also were seen as impediments to attending training programs.

Preferred topics for training

Table 5 shows the training topics preferred by prevention program managers. They were likely to attend training programs for all the topics that were listed. The highest ranked topic was "how to evaluate the effectiveness of HIV prevention programs." When asked what area of training their CBO needed most (data not shown), the topics that were rated the highest were: "how to evaluate effectiveness of HIV/AIDS prevention programs," "what influences certain kinds of behavior and what causes people to behave in ways that put themselves at risk," and "how to empower/mobilize individuals and communities to prevent HIV/AIDS."

Preferred format for training

Preferred formats for training are listed in Table 6. Workshops were the preferred format with seminars and on-the-job training following in preference, respectively. Audiocassette tapes for self-study and telephone conferencing were the least preferred formats for training.

Differences in training needs and preferences between CDC-funded CBOs and nonCDC-funded CBOs

Table 7 lists the 12 dependent factors measuring the training needs and preferences of CBO program managers and compares the response mean of CDC-funded CBOs with nonCDC-funded CBOs.

Organizational support

The 11-item scale measuring organizational support (see Table 2) was reduced to two underlying variables using factor analysis. The variable *Innovation* measured whether executive directors agreed that as a result of training, the capacity for strategic planning and incorporating public health prevention practices into their current practice would increase and new community ties would be forged. *Maintenance* measured the executive director's perceptions of how training would influence funding opportunities and program maintenance. In a test of reliability using Cronbach's alpha, the two scales scored .82 and .83, respectively.

There was no significant difference between executive directors of CDC-funded CBOs and nonCDC-funded CBOs with respect to *Innovation* ($F = .390$, $p = .533$) and *Maintenance* ($F = .416$, $p = .519$). Executive directors of both categories of CBOs strongly agreed that training could result in new innovations being used by their CBO (total mean = 3.38) and that training also would enhance their program's ability to obtain funding (total mean = 3.39), thus enhancing program longevity and effectiveness.

Benefits of training

Factor analysis reduced the 13-item scale measuring the benefits of attending a training program (see

Table 3) to two underlying variables. The first variable, *Personal Rewards*, measured how program managers would benefit personally from training. Variable ingredients included tangible benefits such as certification of training and documentation in a personnel file and intangible benefits of training such as clarifying personal reasons for working in HIV/AIDS prevention. The second variable, *Stimulation*, measured the opportunities to network and exchange ideas with other prevention program managers and the benefits of those exchanges, including the overall improvement of the CBO. Scale reliability scores for each factor were .83 and .77, respectively.

There was no difference between the program managers of CDC-funded and nonCDC-funded CBOs with respect to *Personal Rewards* (F = .996, p = .319). Program managers of CDC-funded and nonCDC-funded CBOs felt these incentives were only somewhat important in influencing their decision to attend training (total mean = 2.48). More importantly, program managers felt that having the opportunity to meet with their peers was more of an incentive to attend a training than personal rewards (*Stimulation* total mean = 3.56). There was no difference between the two categories of CBOs when examining *Stimulation* (F = .071, p = .790).

Barriers to training

Factor analysis reduced the 12-item scale measuring barriers to training to three variables. The first variable, *Separation*, measured feelings about being away from work and home in order to attend a training program. Variable components included being away too long from their job and not having anyone to replace them or take over their assigned activities while they were away. Paid leave was also an issue considered as well as being away from home too long. The inter-item coefficient for this scale was a Cronbach's alpha of .66.

The second factor to emerge from the barrier scale was *Convenience*. This factor measured how convenient a proposed training format would be for program managers if it included having to access technology such as computerized training courses and down-link sites for satellite conferencing. This factor also included the item measuring a program manager's ability to work and do a self-study course. Scale reliability score for this factor was .75.

The last factor in barriers to training was *Application*. This factor measured how applicable new knowledge and skills gained through training would be to their current prevention practice. Items comprising this factor included not earning sufficient rewards for attending training feeling that even if new information was acquired, it would not get used by their CBO, and generally believing that a training program on prevention would not be applicable to their current work.

Scale reliability score for application was .55. It should be noted that although the reliability scores from two factors of the barrier score, *Separation* and *Application*, had lower than preferred inter-item coefficients (< .70 Cronbach's alpha), it was determined by the authors that each scale did represent a barrier of interest and therefore both were retained.

The strongest barrier to attending a training program was *Separation* (total mean = 2.65). There was no difference between CDC-funded CBOs and nonCDC-funded CBOs (F = 3.55, p = .061) as both groups agreed *Separation* would keep them from attending prevention training. Neither *Convenience* (total mean = 2.09) nor *Application* were strong deterrents to attending training and again there was no difference between the two categories of CBOs (F = .716, p = .398; F = .416, p = .519, respectively).

Preferred topics

Factor analysis reduced the list of preferred topics for training to just one factor, *Topics* (Cronbach's alpha = .92). As noted in Table 5, all of the suggested topics were met with enthusiasm. Overall mean score for *Topics* was 3.41. There was no difference between CDC-funded CBOs and nonCDC-funded CBOs (F = .008, p = .931).

Preferred formats

The 13-item scale measuring program managers' preferred format for a training program (see Table 6) was reduced to two factors using factor analysis. The two factors to emerge were *Distant* and *Personal Interaction*. *Distant* accounted for distant learning formats (Cronbach's alpha = .83) and *Personal Interaction* measured more face-to-face formats for training such as workshops, seminars, classroom study, and on-the-job training (Cronbach's alpha = .67).

Program managers strongly preferred face-to-face training (total mean = 3.26) over distance-based learning (total mean = 2.52). This preference was consistent across both categories of CBOs and no difference in the strength of their preferences was found (F = .044, p = .834; F = .113, p = .737, respectively).

Preferred educational level and length of training

Two additional measurements that were important to determining preferences for training were single-item questions and did not require factor analysis. One question asked program managers at what level of education courses should be offered. They were extended three choices for their preferred educational level of coursework: 1 = high school, 2 = college/undergraduate, and 3 = graduate. Respondents specified a preference for courses that were at least at the college level, perhaps slightly higher (total mean = 2.23). There was no difference between CDC funded CBOs and nonCDC-funded CBOs (F = 1.10, p = .843).

Executive directors were polled for their preference on how many consecutive days at any one time a program manager could be absent from work to attend training. Choices included: 1 = 1–3 days; 2 = 4–7 days; 3 = 8–14 days; 4 = 15–30 days; 5 = 31–6 days; 6 = duration not a factor. The total mean score for preferred length of training was 1.93. Executive directors, while enthusiastic about training, preferred their program managers to be away from work for no more than seven days at any one time. There was no difference between CDC-funded CBOs and nonCDC-funded CBOs (F = 1.13, p = .288).

Conclusion and Discussion

Research findings suggest that training is a viable avenue to pursue in helping CBOs improve their capacity to deliver effective HIV/AIDS prevention programs. The benefits of attending a training program are multiple while the barriers to attending are few. Although previous research indicated that HIV prevention staff did not view training as an important source of new information,[12] the results of this survey showed that a significant number of CBO program managers would participate in a training program. The results also indicated that training is needed in multiple areas of public health including strategic management, evaluation, program design, needs assessment, behavioral science, empowerment, advocacy, creating of community capacity to problem solve, collaboration, and cost-analysis. There were no differences in training preferences and needs between CDC-funded and nonCDC-funded CBOs, indicating that a single model for training would serve the needs of both groups.

An interesting result that did emerge from this study that runs contrary to models of training currently being developed in other areas of public health is the lack of preference for distance-based learning. Distance learning quickly is becoming a preferred format in education and training, yet CBO program managers seemed resistant to using the Internet or satellite-based approaches. Even though more than 90 percent of the responding CBOs reported having a computer and 83 percent had modems, only 69 percent had access to the Internet (data not shown). Understanding why program managers oppose using this kind of training format needs further exploration. It could be a matter of comfort level—they are more familiar with traditional training formats and therefore prefer them to other more innovative options. But because the Internet is fast becoming a resource for vast amounts of information, an argument can be made for the idea that improving one's ability to navigate the Web and negotiate electronic mail (e-mail) enhances organizational capacity and HIV prevention efforts. While program managers were quite emphatic about their preference for hands-on, face-to-face training that would allow for an active exchange of ideas and experiences among trainees, the authors believe that a combination of classroom and distance learning provides the best format for instruction because it combines the program managers' stated preference for face-to-face formats with a mechanism for increasing interaction and continued learning between scheduled training sessions.

The intensity of need, given the number of topics for which program managers expressed a desire, will require multiple days for training. But executive directors do not want to have their program managers absent from work for more than seven days at any one time. This suggests that training should occur over several weeks with the training weeks separated by a period of time during which the program managers are back working in their CBOs. Distance learning could be introduced as a means to keep program managers connected to the training program while they are back at work. Actual course work need not be conducted online but discussion board and chat rooms could be used as a way to keep training participants in touch with the program and each other. This would provide a very non-threatening introduction to distance learning for program managers hesitant to participate in distance-based formats.

The willingness of the CDC to continue financially supporting community efforts in HIV prevention recognizes the contribution CBOs have made to the national effort to control the spread of HIV. Now regarded as major partners in public health disease prevention, CBOs soon may be rewarded with a national model for training to help increase their capacity to prevent disease with even greater precision. A training experience that emphasizes strategic management skills and the practice of public health prevention will enhance the individual and organizational capacities of CBOs to deliver more effective and efficient HIV prevention programs. In doing so, the entire national effort to minimize the spread of HIV is strengthened.

REFERENCES

1. Centers for Disease Control and Prevention, *Community-Based Human Immunodeficiency Virus (HIV) Prevention Projects*. Program Announcement 704. Atlanta: Centers for Disease Control and Prevention, 1997.
2. M.E. Bailey, "Community-Based Organizations and CDC as Partners in HIV Education and Prevention," *Public Health Reports* 106, no. 6 (1991): 702–707.
3. R.O. Valdiserri, et al., "Structuring HIV Prevention Service Delivery Systems on the Basic Social Science Theory," *Journal of Community Health* 17, no. 5 (1992): 259–269.
4. J.A. Kelly, et al., "Psychological Interventions To Prevent HIV Infection Are Urgently Needed. New Priorities for Behavioral Research in the Second Decade of AIDS," *American Psychologist* 48, no. 19 (1993): 1023–1034.
5. D.R. Holtgrave, et al., "An Overview of the Effectiveness and Efficiency of HIV Prevention Programs," *Public Health Reports* 110, no. 2 (1995): 134–146.
6. J. Curran, "Bridging the Gap between Behavioral Science and Public Health Practice in HIV Prevention," *Public Health Reports* 111, suppl. 1 (1996): 3–4.
7. L.C. Leviton and K. O'Reilly, "Adaptation of Behavioral Theory to CDC's HIV Prevention Research: Experience at the Centers for Disease Control and Prevention," *Public Health Reports* 111, suppl. 1 (1996): 11–17.
8. C. Sparks, et al., *Summary Report of Existing Information Pertaining to Needs for Behavioral Science Expertise in HIV Prevention Community Planning Groups*. Washington, DC: American Psychological Association Office on AIDS, 1996.
9. A. DeGroff, "From Research to the Front Lines," in *Proceedings of the XI International Conference on AIDS*. Vancouver, BC: XI International Conference on AIDS Society, 1996.
10. E. Goldstein, et al., "Sources of Information for HIV Prevention Program Managers: A National Survey," *AIDS Education and Prevention* 10, no. 1 (1998): 63–74.
11. T. Baranowski, et al., "How Individuals, Environments, and Health Behavior Interact," in *Health Behaviors and Health Education: Theory, Research, and Practice*, 2d ed., ed. K. Glanz, et al. San Francisco: Jossey-Bass, 1997.
12. D.A. Dillman, *Mail and Telephone Surveys: The Total Design Method*. New York: John Wiley & Sons, 1978.